Praise for *Insomnia Doc's Guide to...*

"Dr. Casey provides valuable information and tangible tips on improving sleep. She breaks things down in an easy-to-understand way and does so with humor. She makes learning about sleep into something you'll look forward to."

—Janelle Hettick, LMSW, mental health therapist and speaker

"Dr. Kristen Casey continuously explains the process of sleep and how to improve sleep hygiene in tangible, digestible ways that all of us can incorporate into our hectic lives."

—Dr. Justin Puder (@amoderntherapist), licensed clinical psychologist

"(1) This is a book that you want to have on your bedside table when your awake at 3 a.m. because it for sure is going to help you fall asleep; (2) Dr. Casey has found a way to take a topic that is rooted in science and biology with terminology that only those with an interest would get, but has created a book that breaks everything down in and informative and relatable way (even with a few jokes here and there) that actually makes you want to learn about sleep instead of making you feel like you are ten years old again with your mom yelling from your doorway telling you to go to bed."

—Kristen Gingrich (@notyouraveragethrpst), LCSW, CADC, CCS

"Dr. Casey is my #1 recommendation for qualified sleep help! Her presence on social media has helped so many find the peace they need, and I'm glad that we have gotten to work together. If you're looking for an easy-to-understand, frustration-free guide to getting your sleep back on track, THIS IS IT!"

—Jesse Lyon (@LyonMentalHealth), MS, CCHt, LMHC,
QS. Chief Dream Scientist at DreamApp

"Dr. Kristen's knowledge and passion for insomnia is evident in her book as she breaks down the research on sleep and insomnia and presents it in an authentic, digestible manner. She is inclusive in her work, provides helpful suggestions to readers, and will make you laugh as she shares her unfiltered thoughts and experiences about sleep, as both an expert in the field and a human being that has struggled with sleep just like the rest of us."

—Jessica Rabon, PhD, licensed psychologist

INSOMNIA DOC'S GUIDE TO RESTFUL SLEEP

remedies for insomnia
and tips for good sleep health

DR. KRISTEN CASEY

Licensed Clinical Psychologist

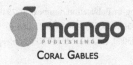

mango
PUBLISHING

CORAL GABLES

Cover Design: Morgane Leoni
Layout & Design: Roberto Núñez

For permission requests, please contact the publisher at:
Mango Publishing Group
2850 S Douglas Road, 2nd Floor
Coral Gables, FL 33134 USA
info@mango.bz

For special orders, quantity sales, course adoptions and corporate sales, please email the publisher at sales@mango.bz. For trade and wholesale sales, please contact Ingram Publisher Services at customer.service@ingramcontent.com or +1.800.509.4887.

Insomnia Doc's Guide to Restful Sleep: Remedies for Insomnia and Tips for Good Sleep Health

Library of Congress Cataloging-in-Publication number: 2022948266
ISBN: (print) 978-1-68481-065-9, (ebook) 978-1-68481-066-6
BISAC category code: HEA043000, HEALTH & FITNESS / Sleep

Printed in the United States of America

David, you inspired me to go on every adventure, especially this one. Your unwavering encouragement, positivity, and support have made all the difference.

Table of Contents

Chapter 1

HOW I (UNEXPECTEDLY) FELL IN LOVE WITH SLEEP

I'm sure you're wondering, "How on earth did you get involved in sleep stuff?" Frankly, I wasn't expecting to become a psychologist, let alone help people with their insomnia. Ironically, I struggled with sleep difficulties in the past but never cared about my sleep health at all. Sleep difficulties also run in my family. My brother was a night owl who would stay up all night to get work done and sleep during the day. I never got a full night of quality sleep because of my work. Honestly, my poor sleep health wasn't on my radar because I was focused on surviving life. I was working through trauma, managing rotating shifts as an EMT, and trying to reconnect with myself to be a better person.

Let's travel back in time to before Kristen was Dr. Casey. It's important for you to know how I relate to the insomnia struggle. But before this, let's talk about the elephant in the room.

The Elephant in the Room

The first elephant is that I will curse and use a lot of humor and weird analogies in this book. It's fun to learn about sleep; it's less fun to read academic articles about it. I've read them and find myself researching sleep pretty often, so I'll take all that information and make it more digestible. The second elephant in the room is how the hell some random person from New York City (me) escaped the rat race and hustle to work on insomnia. Life is a wild ride.

We know some people get into the mental health field to learn more about themselves. In hindsight, I wasn't interested in the mental health field yet; I was trying to figure out how life worked and if my life was normal. I'm sure this is a collective thought for most of us. I've had my struggles, just like everyone else. I decided to write this book because I noticed that a lot of sleep information is either much too basic (only focuses on sleep hygiene) or super jargoned and academic (absolutely love this and it has a place, but it might make some information inaccessible to laypeople). So, I'm hoping to strike a balance here. You might see me explain concepts in simple terms but with enough detail to know the inner workings of sleep.

It's important for you to have somewhat of an idea of who I am and where I've come from so you can identify if this book is a safe space. Of course, it's my intention that this is a safe space for you to learn about and prioritize your sleep, but it's ultimately up to you to decide if it is. The reader-author connection is kinda like developing the patient-provider rapport in therapy:

> **Without trust or understanding, it's hard to see any growth or progress.**

If you think your therapist doesn't hear or see you, it's hard for you to want to learn from them or share things with them. The same goes for reading a book about mental well-being; knowing the author's intentions is essential.

I have the credentials that any well-versed clinical psychologist would have. I received my Doctor of Psychology (PsyD) degree from Midwestern University in Arizona, an APA-accredited program. The American Psychological Association (APA) regulates and accredits certain psychology training programs to ensure they meet certain standards. I completed an APA-accredited internship and optional postdoctoral fellowship at the Department of Veterans Affairs (VA), my top choice for training.

I was trained in evidence-based psychotherapy and evaluation/assessments. It came naturally to me and was incredibly fun to learn. But the training was rigorous and difficult. I remember some nights I'd stay up late and cry, wondering if it was all worth it. I sacrificed so much for this degree, it almost cost me my relationship at one point. It challenged me to work with people I never thought I'd ever come into contact with. I knew there was a lot to learn, so I always tried to be one step ahead, defending my dissertation early or getting licensed earlier than others. But that doesn't make me better; it lets you know that I was so anxious and concerned about succeeding that I did everything in my power to ensure I was as well-trained as possible. In hindsight, I wish I had a little more chill.

I got licensed in two states and then extended this license to twenty-eight states with the help of The Psychology Interjurisdictional Compact (PSYPACT), an agreement that helps psychologists practice telehealth across state lines to increase access to mental healthcare services. I took my training seriously and pride myself on always valuing ethics and professionalism in the therapy room and when I conduct assessments. I always felt a little more edgy and nontraditional looking for a psychologist, so I tried my best to fit in.

This sounds great, right? A good training program and everything checks out. Although I have credentials and I'm a well-trained psychologist, not all psychologists have the same lived experiences, clinical training, or lens that they view the world. This affects the way that we treat clients. It is critical to acknowledge this for the people we treat and the information we put out for the world to see.

It's my goal to make this book as inclusive as possible while also telling you, yes, I am still learning. We are all learning about other cultures and ways of existing, and I say this because everyone handles stress differently, and stress affects our sleep. I took some time to reflect on this before writing this book, and I hope to incorporate these factors into the chapters. So, if your life is different from mine (or providers who look like me), know that I see you and the fact that we may be different.

Insomnia, Diversity, and Whiteness

When I started writing this book I was like, "Yeah, this will be easy." [insert frantic research meme here] Then I started to think about stress and how it affects people differently. It took me a while to figure out how to incorporate this, and I figured I'd do research to figure out how to make an insomnia book easy to read but to feel inclusive for people who don't fit the societal norm.

So, it's impossible to talk about sleep health without also talking about diversity. Stress for someone affluent looks different from stress for someone who doesn't know when their next meal is. Stress is different for a Black woman in a corporate room full of white men and women. It's different for someone paralyzed from the waist down who needs help getting in and out of bed each night. It's different for a trans woman in a room full of cis women and men. My point isn't to compare life experiences but to acknowledge that there are inherent differences in experiences, even when we talk about stress.

I consider that not everyone can fix their stress by fixing their thoughts (which might be loosely based on a Cognitive Behavioral Therapy [CBT] model) because many of these stressful situations are out of their control and impact their survival experiences. Yes, we can think about them differently, but it doesn't change the experience of race-related stress, misogyny in the workplace, or feeling inherently undervalued by society because your disability stops you from working a full-time job. So, blindly telling someone to engage in scheduled worry time or to change their thoughts doesn't change how they experience life. It might invalidate their experience further, so we have to be sensitive to this as we discuss strategies for reducing stress as it relates to sleep health.

That being said, I'm a white, able-bodied, bisexual cisgender woman. Not everyone experiences life in this way. There are inherent privileges to living life from this perspective and it's important to note that I've benefited from these privileges in many ways, regardless of if I acknowledge this and work toward reducing my inherent biases. Although insomnia is a bitch sometimes, insomnia for a white person looks different compared to insomnia for a person of color. Now I know you might be thinking, "Wait, what's the point of saying this? Isn't this a book about insomnia?"

Yes, it is. And the book isn't worth writing (in my opinion) if we don't acknowledge systemic issues that deter people from receiving help or sleep education. **Consequently, everyone will take these sleep tips differently based on their unique situations.** I mean, sheeeesh, there are plenty of barriers to gaining this information in the first place, which starts with us as providers. The mental healthcare system is kind of fucked. It needs to be more accessible in several ways, and sometimes providers are at a loss with whatever we try to do. Sometimes this is out of our control. Yet, what we providers can control are the way we interact with people from other cultures, the knowledge we have of people that are different from us, a deep desire to attempt to understand what different ways of living might be like, actively engaging in policy change by signing petitions, being actively anti-racist, anti-homophobic, or anti-transphobic, knowing that we don't know it all, and actively taking a stance against white supremacy and misogyny, etc. Yes, even when we treat someone with plain ol' insomnia.

It starts (at a bare minimum) with taking ownership of how these systems have benefited the majority of the population and with having a genuine desire to reach populations that desperately need our help. Then, it is a lifelong journey to ensure that we are contributing to these systems in the ways we can and checking ourselves along the way. We can't talk about mental health and sleep without also talking about stress because stress keeps people up at night. Knowing the type of stress and its impact is incredibly important. For example, if a BIPOC reader doesn't feel seen or heard (at a bare minimum, bar is in the basement, y'all), they may not think these sleep tips apply to them. It's no surprise that minority voices desperately want (and deserve) culturally competent education materials and mental health treatment and can often be in the medical room with a provider who is oblivious to the idea of systemic oppression and how that relates to their insomnia symptoms.

We are gradually making changes like updating academic curriculum, promoting inclusivity, and requiring continuing education for cultural competency. Books should speak to this in the beginning and include that this is an inherent problem we are trying to fix. Otherwise, minority readers may have intentions of learning about insomnia, yet their lifestyles aren't being included in the text and may think, "What's the point of even reading the book then?" **It's helpful to know if a book will apply to you before you dedicate your time to reading it.**

Another question you might have is, "Shouldn't a minority who has experienced sleep issues be writing this book?" Ideally, yes. It would be incredible to lift up minority voices in the insomnia world. It's a catch-22 here because that also lets people with privilege off the hook. Why? Because now they don't have to talk about it (which is part of the problem). It's important for people with privilege to take accountability and realize that turning a blind eye and only having discussions with people who look similar to them only makes the problem worse, especially within the context of mental well-being and sleep health. I notice that many white providers occupy the sleep education realm, and I'm one of them. Acknowledging this is crucial to welcome providers from other cultures to occupy this space, too.

And yeah, white, able-bodied, cisgender providers or educators might feel fearful of saying/writing the right thing, or might be scared about acknowledging their privilege, or might not believe they have privilege to begin with (let me throw my laptop across the room; I hate that I even had to write that). That is the problem within itself. We have to start showing up to have these conversations with the opportunity to receive corrective feedback to know if what we are doing is helpful or not. This is where it starts; there is always more work to do.

Let's Get Uncomfortable

If you're cringing as you read this, it might resonate [insert white fragility references here], just know I was also there at one point. I'm not ashamed to admit that I was taught that privilege didn't exist and everything is a choice in life. I still have a lot to learn, but I realized that this way of thinking serves nobody besides white people and the patriarchy. And fuck the patriarchy, honestly.

So, if we get a little uncomfortable acknowledging some privilege, especially while providing insomnia and mental health education, it's still not as terrible as having to experience discrimination based on how you look, where you come from, or your culture/life values, and then educate people on how to treat you fairly. I say all this to let you know that this is where I'm coming from. And to my friends who acknowledge their privilege and take steps to have these conversations: let's meet up and chat about it. I'm all ears.

The field of psychology is becoming more diverse, yet I noticed that sleep education may sometimes stem from cis white heterosexual norms. Not everyone can purchase super comfy sheets or pillows or have a completely quiet room to sleep in. And some people do have this ability. Not knocking you for wanting comfy sheets; I get it. Providing education solely from this perspective without focusing on inclusivity or identifying ways to include other lifestyles can be harmful. It also creates barriers for minorities to have access to sleep health information, let alone implement some helpful strategies.

I also recognize that not everyone can have time and space to focus on their sleep health. If you're worried about how to pay your bills, or when your next meal is, trying to prioritize sleep will be a tough sell. Like other providers, I like to use a harm-reduction approach when it comes to sleep health. This means that we use practical strategies to meet the person where they are, even if they don't meet the mold of generalized standards. So, if an insomnia protocol suggests waking up at the same time each day, that might not be possible for everyone. So, we try to find consistency for this person in other ways, such as having the same waking routine or choosing certain shifts on certain days. Instead of forcing the person into a box of consistency that isn't realistic for them, we work together to find what works for them. In other words, we focus on increasing quality even in the smallest ways.

As you can see, there might be several limitations and the traditional ways of working on sleep that might not be so helpful for every person. This is why it's important for me to acknowledge that not everyone meets the norms when it comes to stress, bed partners, sleep arrangements, sleep values, and more. By reading this book, the goal is to meet you where you are and figure out how to make sleep a little better in small steps. So, small steps might be all we have right now, and it's better than not helping yourself at all. Prioritizing your sleep not only helps you, but it also helps the rest of the world because your relationship with yourself affects all others. Sleep affects your mental health, and this impacts how you experience the world.

I hope to create space for different lived experiences and meet people where they are within the context of these limitations so that you can make even small changes that will help your sleep dramatically. If you feel like the vibe checks out, keep reading so we can chat about where this all began. I'm going to get a little vulnerable with you because fuck it, why not. I'll be six feet under one day so we may as well go all in!

Where It All Began

My Insomnia Roots

You'll probably relate to this, which is why I needed to include it in this book. So, my life was a bit unstable from childhood until I started grad school, and I noticed that my mood was mostly dictated by those around me. I was a self-proclaimed empath, so to speak. Do you take on the emotions of people around you? Do you feel responsible for making them okay or ensuring they're having a good time? Yeah, same here. This shit kept me up at night.

I was always waiting for someone around me to tell me how to feel or to reassure me that everything was okay. It was difficult to figure out how I truly felt when I was constantly making sure everyone around me was okay. I had an innate sense of wanting to help others, probably to a detriment, because I lost sight of who I was for a while. When I look back on my life, I realized there's a reason for this. I can easily blame other people or my circumstances. I chalk it up to a perfect storm of my family going through tough experiences (like most of us), experiencing intense insomnia, having a deep desire to stop generational cycles, truly wanting to connect with others on a raw level, some spiritual awakenings, caring about the greater good of society, and figuring out how I can have some sense of purpose.

I never thought I would say this out loud, let alone write it in a book, but my parents did their best at the time—trying to survive their generational trauma cycles and parenting to the best of their ability, all while trying to live outside of the box. Sleep wasn't a priority in my family, ever. For legal and personal reasons, I'm only going to discuss certain aspects of my life within the context of this book but I figured I would speak as much as I could about how insomnia has impacted my life without jeopardizing my family's privacy. Insomnia may stem from trauma, and trauma has many layers. In this case, it's worth sharing generalities with you because it's a good example of how it makes insomnia symptoms worse. You can love your family so much *and* acknowledge that your upbringing messed you up. My family would agree that their upbringing messed them up too.

I Mastered Survival Mode, but It Kept Me Up at Night

I was always an anxious kid, kinda like you. Aside from that, we know that collective family trauma can change us in some way. For me, the unpredictability of my childhood kept me up at night. All. Friggen. Night. I'm sure you can relate if you've been through some stuff in childhood. At the time, I didn't realize this stress technically contributed to my insomnia. I thought it was normal.

I remember laying in my bed at night, thinking about everything in my life and how I could have maybe changed things or done things differently. I also thought a lot about the things that were outside of my control. Looking back, all of these life circumstances fueled my insomnia. **What you don't process keeps you up at night, which includes your hopes, fears, dreams, lost opportunities, trauma, and things you leave unsaid.**

My family and I lived parallel lives without truly connecting. And nobody ever asked me, "What's keeping you up at night?" Now, this is something I ask all of my clients. So, if someone blindly told me to engage in sleep hygiene, I'd probably laugh and be like, "Okay, but will that fix years of trauma or what?" There's more to it than that, which is why this book might be helpful for you.

How This Relates to Insomnia

Buckle up, bestie. We're diving right in here. Most of what I just talked about falls under the predisposing factors for insomnia. It's part of the 3p Model introduced by Spielman and colleagues in 1987.[1] The three P's are predisposing, precipitating, and perpetuating factors, which all contribute to insomnia.

---

1   Spielman, A. J., Caruso, L. S., and Glovinsky, P. B. (1987). A behavioral perspective on insomnia treatment. *Psychiatric Clinics of North America, 10*(4), 541-553.

Predisposing factors are long-lasting issues that contribute to the
onset and maintenance of insomnia, such as family history of trauma,
genetic predispositions, or dispositional traits that we're born with,
which occur before insomnia becomes a real issue. Early intervention
models for insomnia focus on these factors, the ones that you're not
expecting to become an issue or even contribute to sleep issues in the
first place. These don't usually contribute to severe insomnia, but
when combined with precipitating and perpetuating factors, that does
happen.[2] It's that combo effect that hits differently.

Some of what I talked about falls under precipitating factors.
Precipitating factors are certain events that lead to (precipitate) sleep
problems, such as experiencing an unsettling divorce or losing a job
that initiates poor sleep onset. Multiple events or recurrent situations
can contribute to the manifestation of insomnia. Finally, perpetuating
factors. Yep, the big daddy of them all, the ones we can control more
than the other two P's. Sometimes precipitating factors resolve
themselves, but we maintain our insomnia symptoms by engaging in
behaviors that contribute to poor sleep, such as perpetuating factors,
like unhelpful thinking patterns or maladaptive coping patterns such
as substance use.

I'm sure you can come up with ideas of how predisposing,
precipitating, and perpetuating factors have contributed to your
insomnia. For example, Black individuals are twice as likely to
experience insomnia symptoms compared to whites.[3] Is this because
of something genetic (e.g., predisposing)? Is it because of one event of
race-related stress (e.g., precipitating factor)? Or can it be the constant

2   Wright, C. D., Tiani, A. G., Billingsley, A. L., Steinman, S. A., Larkin, K. T., and McNeil, D. W. (2019).
     A framework for understanding the role of psychological processes in disease development,
     maintenance, and treatment: The 3P-Disease Model. *Frontiers in Psychology*, *10*(2498).

3   Kingsbury, J. H., Buxton, O. M., and Emmons, K. M. (2013). Sleep and its relationship to racial and
     ethnic disparities in cardiovascular disease. *Current Cardiovascular Risk Reports*, *7*(5), 387-394.

race-related systemic stress that Black Americans experience every day (e.g., perpetuating)?

Everyone has a different starting line, so I encourage my clients to look at their insomnia as unique because there are many different factors to consider. Your life is different from your neighbor's, your friend's, or even your family member's. I had to do the same thing because it seemed like everyone around me was sleeping and I was awake AF at night.

The Change

Back to our timeline: I managed to graduate high school, but I had no direction and still wasn't sleeping well. I was sick of myself, sick of not being able to sleep at night either. The true change was my experience in the ambulance, which coincidentally made my insomnia way worse. I joined the first aid squad, became an EMT, and volunteered a ton of my time. Probably too much time. It felt like a calling, I fell in love with it. If I wasn't in school or working, I was on the rig. I responded to natural disasters and car accidents, did a ton of CPR, saw a lot of blood, and gave a lot of good and bad news to people.

I still wasn't thinking about my sleep. In fact, I was sleeping even less. At this point, I had experienced poor sleep for over ten years, and I wasn't even twenty years old when I joined the first aid squad.

Throughout my time in the ambulance, my insomnia became noticeably worse. Who knew that working all day and staying up all night to answer calls in the middle of the night is a for-sure way to wreck your circadian rhythm? On night shift, I would sleep in my bed and my pager would wake me up in the middle of the night. I started to get triggered by my bed because I knew I would be woken up at some point. Once the pager went off, we didn't know what we were getting into because dispatchers gave us limited information. Not their fault but it got you thinking about what you'd see. I'd make it to the scene, hope people lived, and come back home to sit and think.

I'm sure you've also felt this in some way, knowing that a thought or environmental circumstance will wake you up, even if you try hard to sleep. I think of people living in high crime areas or with little ones who wake them up at weird hours throughout the night.

I'd get home, sit on the side of my bed, and think. It seemed like I would think about stuff for endless hours. Time didn't seem to make sense and I was conscious of my thoughts. Think about the situation, think about what I could have done better, think about how to show up differently to be more effective. I didn't care though; I was doing what I loved.

All the while, I finished my bachelor's in New Jersey and randomly moved to Arizona for some change. I was so stressed out because I had no idea where I was going or what to do; I just knew I didn't want to spend another day in New Jersey. Sorry, friends, it just wasn't my kind of party. But this wasn't a foreign feeling, dealing with the unpredictability. Once I got to Arizona, I applied to clinical psychology doctorate programs there. I was like, *What the hell, I didn't think I'd make it this far, so let's see what happens.* At this point, I noticed my sleep issues a little more.

I Discovered That Sleep Was Part of the Psychology World

Who knew? I didn't think sleep was anything we'd ever talk about in graduate school. I went to an interview for a PsyD program and one of the first questions they asked me was, "What's your 'why'?" I almost broke down in tears, then remained professional and said, "I love helping people and want to be a safe place for people." But what I wanted to say was, "I love holding space for people because I wish someone had held space for me when I was younger. Maybe I would have loved myself sooner or helped myself heal instead of hurting myself in the process, and hope to pay this forward in some way." I remember being *so exhausted* when I answered this question.

Fast-forward, I got into the program. I had dark circles from not sleeping, whereas other people appeared peppy and ready for the day. I also almost felt *too* edgy, like this deep sense that I didn't belong for some reason. Some of my colleagues simply knew they wanted to be psychologists from a young age. And here I was, continuing school because it was one of the only stable factors in my life. I wanted to pay it forward and hoped learning happened as a natural consequence. I was always concerned with the greater outcome of humanity, so I had that going for me. Ironically, I wasn't too attached to the outcome, which in hindsight, was a great mindset to have. If I graduated, it was meant to be. If not, I'd figure it out. Looking back, it was the challenge I desperately needed. I was not only challenged clinically and academically, but I also unexpectedly fell in love with sleep and diversity.

There's more that happened before my sleep health improved. One of the consequences of graduate school was that I went to therapy. My guardian angels were probably up there saying, "Goddamn, this trainwreck *finally* made it to therapy!" I'm not super religious, but if I was, I imagine this would be the scene. It was almost like divine intervention.

I wanted to sit in a chair and get uncomfortable with my therapist if I wanted my clients to do this. My sole purpose for doing this was to become a good therapist and psychologist. Our program didn't require it. I found a therapist that was so chill, yet professional. She was covered in tattoos, was super professional and ethical, but always laughed at my dark humor (then would ask me to unpack it, of course). She challenged me, yet I could tell she truly cared about me. She saw me; I trusted her. I told her stuff that I never told anybody, the deep stuff. You ever have something that happened to you and you're like *Yeah, I'm never telling* anybody *about this shit*? Yeah, I thought that was me until I met my therapist. I told her what was keeping me up at night. *Finally* somebody asked me that question.

Something that never went away was that burning passion for holding space for people. I didn't care if it was raw and sad or happy and exciting. The most challenging part of this entire thing was my clinical internship. It was so challenging that I didn't think I would make it at one point. It also helped me learn about people that were different from me. I started yelling at older white men to stop being misogynistic and yelled at myself for not challenging my privilege sooner. **This internship was also the pivotal moment when I started caring about my sleep.** But there were a few clinical experiences before that that made my insomnia worse before it got better.

The Clinical Internship That Changed My View on Sleep

Okay, nobody gets excited about sleep randomly, right? Wrong. This internship helped me see that there's a whole community of people who give a shit about other people's sleep. It was fascinating.

Clinical psychology internships are competitive, and I've never been good at competitions. I love when everyone wins or if there is space for everyone. I woke up on match day hungover after two hours of sleep to learn that I matched to my top site, the Department of Veterans Affairs (VA). I was like, *Holy shit; how does the VA want someone like me?* I still couldn't believe it. I thought they had made a mistake. I felt like I was always trying to push it away and it held me back. But I didn't realize these experiences would be invaluable in helping me learn more about other people as a psychologist. I later learned that these lived experiences are *gold* if you fuel them into your clinical practice in the right way. The VA is known for excellent training for psychologists. It's a dream job for most people. I got there, and they were like, "Kristen! So honored to have you." I still couldn't figure out what they saw in me. Over time, I gained confidence but remembered to stay humble because it's impossible to know everything. I had no idea that I would focus so much on sleep. I thought I would retire as a psychologist in an inpatient unit somewhere because I was used to the crisis on the ambulance (and during my childhood, hehe).

The training was way different than I expected. In my grad program, we talked about diversity, but not quite like this. These training sessions were next level; they reinforced that white fragility is something to be challenged, even when you treat someone with insomnia. This solidified my desire to learn more about how I can show up differently for people of color and other women. I realized that sleep was most likely different for marginalized communities, which would affect how we provide treatment to certain populations. There was *always something* new to learn. I learned that treatment for different groups of people should look different, even if you're using an evidence-based manual.

I honestly thought that sleep was so basic, dull, and bland. When you treat trauma, you have to keep diversity in mind, right? Well, it's just as important when you work with insomnia. I wasn't exactly jazzed about providing this treatment from the outset.

The Required Rotation That Showed Me Sleep Is Life

This internship taught me a lot, challenged my beliefs, and allowed me to help veterans. Learning how to balance being there for the client but being myself all the while, I was exhausted. I assisted with a transgender support group and fell in love with helping this population. I also had the opportunity to cofacilitate a Dialectical Behavior Therapy (DBT) skills group, which I also loved. I stayed up late reading the protocols and watching videos about how to implement the skills in a professional but human way. I didn't want to be a robot, but I wanted to use this knowledge to guide regular conversations. I learned these protocols for helping people through trauma, anxiety, and depression and helped them enhance life fulfillment. I would get so excited when veterans showed up for therapy. I was honored to do evaluations and assessments. I was glad people wanted to connect with me. Whether it was personal or professional, connection meant the world to me. What's not to love? Then, the shitshow began.

There was this required rotation when I worked in primary care. This rotation sent me into a spiral, in a good way. A Cognitive Behavioral Therapy for Insomnia (CBT-I) group. I was like *Fuck, I don't want to do this at all.* I knew nothing about sleep health. I struggled so badly with insomnia my entire life. How can I teach veterans about sleep when my insomnia dates back to childhood? Then it dawned on me: *Wow, finally, something I dislike about this internship.*

I never talked about my insomnia until this point. I was ashamed, to be honest. I thought aspiring psychologists should have their lives together and be good role models for their clients. Who would trust me if I couldn't sleep at night? I was under the impression that most psychologists and therapists are "blank slates" and that they didn't share anything about themselves with the public (or their clients). We aren't perfect. When I let go of the idea that psychologists have to be perfect replicas of the product of lifelong healing, was the time that I noticed I was more open to the idea of working on my sleep. The more I acknowledged I struggled with sleep, the more I could see the relief in my clients' eyes. They knew they weren't alone.

I had two amazing supervisors who were both into sleep health. Like, not just excited about sleep, but ran sleep groups, offered one-on-one therapy with people about sleep, even if they didn't have room in their schedule, the whole nine yards. I was lost. How the hell was sleep so fun for them? I can barely get five hours of solid sleep per night. They were like drinking some sleep juice or something and I was trying to figure out where to get it. I wanted whatever sleep excitement drugs they were taking.

One of my supervisors was like, "Listen, this is a required rotation; we need you to help with this insomnia group."

"There's no way. Can I do something else? I don't think it fits into my professional goals; it's not something I ever thought of doing."

"More of a reason to try it. See you tomorrow."

Dammit. I didn't want to, but I agreed because who says no to their supervisor when they think something will be good for you? I trusted her. Why was I so resistant to this group? I meditated and realized there was more to this than thinking it was boring.

I didn't know anything about sleep. I was a novice. The only thing I did was set an alarm to wake up in the morning and hoped I had enough energy to sustain me throughout the day. I didn't know how to help people with sleep and didn't know how to help myself, either. I relied on over-the-counter sleep medications when I was struggling.

I didn't have any tools in my toolbox. I had nothing to offer. But I had to remember something: we train to learn, not to know everything. Otherwise, there's no point in putting yourself through an internship.

So, how it works is that you observe the group, help with notes, and then run the group once you feel good about it. *How the hell will I ever feel good about this when my sleep is shit too? Veterans are smart; they'll know I have insomnia, too.* I didn't realize it at the time, but this served me well as a group facilitator.

And you know what? They knew, and we got through it together. They were patient with me as I learned from my supervisor. I decided to do the same treatment on myself as I observed and facilitated with the group. Holy shit, I wasn't expecting this outcome. I was miserable for a few days. Like, exhausted. The most tired I've ever been in my life. I remember I was so tired that I left work early because I wasn't effective. Then, it was like a light switch. It all changed. I felt like I could wake up easier, I was less fatigued, I had a bedtime routine, I woke up to one alarm. What the actual hell?

My sleep wasn't perfect, but it was somewhat predictable. I had more realistic expectations for myself, and I had some choice points to improve my sleep quality if I dipped into my old habits again. I guess that's what we're going for in insomnia treatment. Simultaneously, the veterans in the group were also getting better. I was accustomed to doing longer-term therapy—you know, about twelve to sixteen weeks. This program lasted only six weeks. I had my doubts, but I was shocked that people got better so quickly. Of course, like any program, there were outliers. People who took a little longer to get better, which made sense given their PTSD symptoms. It didn't cure everything, like stress and how society treats veterans, but it reduced symptoms enough for these people to feel like they can function again. **Focusing**

**on their sleep health created space for them to meet themselves
again, and it was a beautiful thing to watch across sessions.**

Then, there's stress. The stuff we were talking about at the beginning
of this book. These veterans experienced stressors that I'd never
even heard of before. Some served in Vietnam; some were people of
color; others had physical disabilities. Some had concussions from
their deployments that posed difficulty with retaining information.
I followed the insomnia protocol to a T. I tried to use what I learned
about diversity and inclusivity within the protocol to meet people
where they were. Stress was different for everyone, and I realized stress
was also the thing that kept me up at night. Stress that was out of my
control. And it was the same for some of them.

"So, how's it going?" my supervisor asked me about the group
in supervision.

"I don't know; maybe I'm starting to like it."

Her eyes lit up. I could tell she was so proud and so excited.

"So do you want to continue doing the group?"

"Yeah, let's give it a whirl."

I ended up facilitating a few CBT-I groups for my internship and the
entire year of my fellowship. I loved it. I researched sleep in my spare
time and looked up research articles about certain sleep protocols.
I was mostly interested in insomnia. I almost hated that I loved it so
much. This is where it all began.

Yeah, I Guess That Sleep Group Was My Favorite

I can't believe I admit this looking back, but that was the best group I ever facilitated. It was challenging, too. We take a ton of sleep data. It's intense; the notes are rigorous. I didn't even care. I noticed myself falling in love with helping people with insomnia. All the while, I was wearing a few different hats in other areas of life, but it all started to improve when my sleep improved. Trauma triggers weren't as bad. I was less irritable. My relationships were more fun. I had more time to do the things I loved rather than stay awake in bed, unable to sleep.

I noticed that insomnia is an issue for a good majority of people. People of all colors, shapes, and sizes. It didn't matter what your upbringing or what you went through; insomnia may have been a symptom of your physical or mental health. That said, I also learned a lot about how insomnia presents differently for people, depending on their color, shape, size, socioeconomic status, cultural/religious background, age, ability level, and more. Learning the basics of helping people with insomnia during my internship, fellowship, and beyond allowed me to refine my skills and learn more about how it affects everyone, not just veterans.

Here We Are Now

I ended up graduating from my APA-accredited doctorate program and passing my internship. I was accepted into the postdoctoral fellowship position in health psychology, where I focused on insomnia, anxiety, and depression in a primary care setting within the VA. I refined my skills for helping those with insomnia; it felt so natural to me. So, I thought I'd retire at the VA and run this CBT-I group forever. Well, that didn't happen. Something even better did.

I was working full-time at a different VA, and I downloaded a social media platform as a joke. I started chatting more about insomnia, and a few videos went viral. I remember one day I woke up with 55,000 new followers after having 10,000 the day before. I thought, *Wow, people really like this information.* People were asking me such great questions, and I ended up creating a community I never knew I needed. I found a newfound sense of purpose and I was reaching a wider audience to talk about sleep, authenticity, and helping white providers learn more about diversity, which was my ultimate goal. This put pressure on me to know my stuff. I started reading more about insomnia and I couldn't believe there was even more to learn.

This online community fostered connection, something I desperately searched for in my life. **This connection wouldn't be possible if I didn't have that required sleep rotation**. If I didn't heal from trauma, lean into my anxiety, and address my insomnia, I'm not sure I'd be here with you writing this book. I also learned so much from people who are academic researchers, sleep medicine experts, and people who do more than CBT-I. Social media opened the door for me to learn more than I ever could, even though I thought that internship had endless information. I'm sure you can relate to this in some way.

At the same time that my social media platforms went viral, my grandma was getting sick. I knew I had to step down from my full-time position at the VA to help out. I was so afraid to leave; it was all I knew. I also didn't want to let go of helping people with their sleep. These psychologists were so generous in training me; how could I leave the VA? Even though my sleep was better, *my soul was tired.* Although I loved the VA, it was a grind at times. There were endless clients and there wasn't enough time to help everyone. It was time for a change.

I decided to leave and go full-time in private practice during the pandemic because I figured people needed more access to mental health care and education, especially for insomnia. I decided to go private pay and open a few free slots for women and minorities. I also do a bunch of other stuff for free, like speaking on podcasts, contributing to articles, and trying to dismantle the patriarchy in my free time. It felt like I could give back in ways that were meaningful to me.

I also knew I wanted to be closer to my family. After all the healing and sleeping I did in Arizona, I knew I was ready to reengage and be closer, but I didn't want to live in Jersey. My partner, David, is from Missouri originally and we decided to move here. The flight to Jersey is three hours rather than almost six, even though I don't visit often. Dave had a huge community in Missouri. I never thought I'd ever live in the Midwest. I thought, *What else is there besides hay and some farms?* Well, a lot more than I expected, but it was more culture shock for me. But, at this point in my life, I'm chasing neutrality and peace rather than excitement and chaos. It's the perfect fit, but I also know I stick out here. I am sleeping wonderfully here, too. There are more sounds of nature and peace than in Arizona and the Big Apple. My neighbor has this cute pig who wakes up at the crack of dawn and oinks; he's basically like a big, cute, pink alarm clock.

Reflections

A few years ago I never thought I'd get out of a mental, physical, and financial dark hole, and now I can't believe life has come full circle. We still struggle, there are still hard times, but for some reason, life feels easier to manage, knowing that I can regain my power in small ways when life becomes tough, especially when I'm not sleeping well. I took the time to be patient with myself and compassionate for my shortcomings, and to accept myself for who I am. I'm not proud of my past mistakes, but they surely gave me some good process points in therapy. **I also realized that sleep was absolutely crucial for my healing. Prioritizing sleep helped me work through the trauma easier and I was showing up as my full potential, and you deserve this too.**

Without these life experiences and graduate school, I'm not sure I would have been prepared for the events that unfolded in 2020, let alone made it this far in life. I feel more equipped to have tough conversations and hold space for others struggling, including my friends and family. I feel more confident in addressing systemic issues that hinder certain people from getting the help they need, especially those struggling with insomnia. I'm always learning more about how to show up more effectively for BIPOC, LGBTQ+, and those with disabilities with regard to sleep issues. I'm challenging my biases and helping other people do the same. I'm open to people telling me I'm doing it wrong, or that I have more to learn. I thank them for telling me because that's how we make changes. I'm having more conversations about white privilege, misogyny, and ableism, in addition to insomnia, with my friends, family, colleagues, and community on social media. This is only the beginning.

Then, I was at another crossroads. I had a successful solo, private telehealth practice helping people with insomnia, anxiety, and gender/sexuality concerns, and I was active on social media. What more could I do? Well, as you know, I've never been relaxed, like, ever, so I kept thinking about what I should do next. Do I open up a lucrative group private practice and hire clinicians to work under me? I know a few clinicians who do that and make some pretty good money. While interviewing some people to work for me, I got approached by a publisher to write this book.

It happened when I was with my friend Loren. She's the friend that I reconnected with after we met on the ambulance a while ago. We stayed close all these years, and she moved to Missouri for a hospital job. I never thought I'd see both of us Jersey gals in the Midwest. We were in the parking lot of the hospital that she was going to interview with, and I looked at my email.

"I got approached by a publisher to write a book."

"Um, what?"

"Yeah, but I don't know because I want to open this group practice and I can't do both."

"Bitch, who says you can't do both?"

She always hypes me up, but I knew I would hate myself if I put any more on my plate. I didn't want to fall back into bad sleep habits *especially* because I was becoming an insomnia expert. I'm big on practicing what I preach. I had social media to push out great content about sleep education, and it reached a decent amount of people. It was more reach than I would ever have in a group practice. My main question/goal was, *How do I get this information to people who need it?* I need to cast the net pretty wide, and seeing individual clients wouldn't send this information out there.

I knew I couldn't do both; I obviously decided to write the book. Group practice would have surely been a great financial move for me; I could pay off all my debt and take care of my family because my parents are getting old. But money isn't the motive. I'm in it for the people, especially the people who don't have the resources to affordably get this information. I'm in it for the people because human connection is the most important thing. I see strangers as my family. I thought this was weird at first, but maybe others feel the same way.

I knew the book wouldn't replace therapy, but it would surely give people some of the education they needed to make good life changes depending on their circumstances. I was thinking people could even gift this book to someone else, pass it down, or share what they've learned. The opportunities are endless, and it fosters more connections. This means more to me than a paycheck. Plus, I'm not going to be worried about how much money I have on my deathbed. I'm going to be worried if I made an impact on people, if they thought I was kind to them, if they got good sleep, and if they felt seen. Nothing else matters.

This isn't just any book about insomnia. **It's a book that makes enhancing your sleep health feel more achievable. It's more than a protocol, more than an academic research article. It incorporates that in it with you in mind, your human self.** I've been there, too, and I'm still in it with you. I still struggle with my sleep. With my life experiences and expertise, I hope you can see this as a safe space to learn more about yourself. The first step starts with your sleep.

Chapter 2

WHY YOU SHOULD CARE ABOUT YOUR SLEEP

So, why should you even care about sleep? I didn't think it was important for a long, long time. I believed that I could sleep when I was dead or that I could catch up on sleep. Spoiler alert: neither of these beliefs is helpful for our sleep health.

I started learning more about what my life might look like without good sleep. I began reading statistics about the lack of quality sleep and freaked out. If I could be honest, it scared the shit out of me. If you want to scare yourself, do a deep dive into what alcohol does to your brain, body, and sleep functions (big yikes!). Lack of quality sleep might have short-term consequences, such as increased sympathetic nervous system arousal (a.k.a. fight-flight-or-freeze response), which releases cortisol, our stress hormone.[4] That straight up doesn't sound good, and it isn't.

We've all heard "in moderation, though!" That can be true. A few nights of poor sleep won't send us into a spiral of poor health outcomes. I'm talking about the everyday struggle for sleep over years. Like, you're waking up in a frenzy and your life feels unorganized because you barely slept and you don't know how you'll get through the day. Picture that for ten, twenty, or even fifty years of your life. It can't be good. Sleep isn't a priority unless we intentionally think about

---

4   Medic, G., Wille, M., and Hemels, M. E. H. (2017). Short-and long-term health consequences of sleep disruption. *Nature and Science of Sleep, 2017*(9), 151–161.

the benefits and how it helps restore our biological processes. Plus, you sound kind of like a buzzkill when you say you want to sleep rather than socialize, work, or do anything fun. That kind of thinking catches up to you eventually.

The truth is, if you don't care about your sleep, nobody else will. It's somewhat of a solo mission once you become an adult and it's so important because small steps in the right direction make a huge difference in our sleep. I know you're probably wondering, "Kristen, why are you so concerned about people's sleep?" Well, I thrive while helping people, but there's a bigger reason here. Buckle up for the most unrealistic story ever. **clicks seatbelt**

Picture if the entire world (every human being and animal) could get restful sleep. Think about how the world would function. We'd be nicer to each other. We'd maybe spend more time with our family. We might remember things that we'd normally forget. People would go the extra mile for others. We might spend a little more time at our jobs because we're rested and our biological needs are met. We might care about the generations that will come after us, long after we're gone. We might take the time to vote on issues that mean the most to us. We might help underprivileged populations so that we can all experience life in a better way. We might make the earth a better place just by the conversations we choose to have. On the other hand, people are exhausted and dredging through life. Some people just want to survive the day. They might not stop and do things for themselves or others.

I care about the collective human experience because this moment—yes, this moment right here while you're reading this sentence—is the only reliable moment you have. You have no idea what will happen after this, even if you planned for it. Tuning into the present moment and collective human experience is important because we are all out here trying to survive all this shit anyway, so we may as well get some quality sleep while doing so. And, if we can enhance our day-to-day life without doing a lot of extra work, and by sleeping a bit more, I think it's worth it. Okay, unbuckle your seatbelt. The imaginary ride is over. Watch your step as you exit.

Obviously, this is *absolutely impossible* with how our world is set up today. People experience homelessness, don't have opportunities for sleep, live below the poverty line, don't have access to basic healthcare, don't know if they'll escape their abusive situations—the list goes on and on. There are people out there who will never have an opportunity to read this book or even consider their sleep. They experience such stress that's outside of their ability to cope effectively, and if I were in their situations, I'd feel the same way.

But here you are, reading this. So you can be the component of change. And it won't directly affect those struggling, but if you are better, then you can make the world better, too. Remember, it starts from within. Although this is impossible, I'm not willing to give up and chalk it up as a loss. We can get better sleep not only for ourselves but for the greater good of the world. Some people don't have this privilege or opportunity, but if we do, then maybe we can have extra brain power or mental space to help them in other ways. So, it's not a direct correlation here, but I think it's worth it. If you can learn something about your sleep and tell someone else about it, that's a win in my book.

The priority for most adults is working, functioning, producing things, and getting things done. Prioritizing sleep doesn't exactly fit into this mold, especially in the United States. Employees that focus on working rather than sleeping are the best employees, right? Yeah, they're also the most exhausted and hate themselves more than they hate the nine-to-five. I'm challenging you to think of sleep as *almost* equally important to doing your job or generally functioning as a human. If your body isn't operating effectively, it'll be difficult to function in your job or enhance your general well-being. And we all want to be a little more fulfilled, right?

Let's dive in and chat about who the hell discovered sleep, what it actually is, and how a lack of quality sleep may impact your overall health.

Who Discovered Sleep?

Sometimes I think about sleep and get lost in a vortex of deep thoughts. Best case scenario, we lay our heads on a fluffy, square-shaped plush thing, shut our eyes, and drift off into the abyss. We're unconscious for a few hours, then magically wake up like nothing ever happened (even though so much happens!). We might have vivid dreams that don't make sense, that aren't technically lived experiences, but they're part of our human experience in general. Our muscles are usually paralyzed so that we don't act out these dreams (atonia during REM sleep),[5] but sometimes we do weird things in our sleep (a.k.a. parasomnias) like engage in sleepwalking (a.k.a. somnambulism) and don't remember it the next day. Make it make sense!

I mean, sleep wasn't invented; it was something we kind of *did*. I wonder how ancient civilizations handled this. Maybe they noticed their friend losing consciousness at night, and they did too, and they couldn't explain it. Did they think they died and came back to life? Did they think it was something they were doing wrong? Did they think it was normal? I have so many questions. Think about the first person

---

5   Mayo Clinic. (2018, Jan. 18). *REM sleep behavior disorder*. https://www.mayoclinic.org/diseases-conditions/rem-sleep-behavior-disorder/symptoms-causes/syc-20352920.

who got brain freeze from ice cream. They were probably *shook*. Anyway, I can imagine that sleep may have been a scary elusive thing, at least it would be for me back then. The milestones within the history of sleep are incredible to think about.

Sleep History: We've Come a Long Way

The first people who discovered the inner workings of sleep were heroes that didn't wear capes at the time. Maybe they wore lab coats, but I'm sure they were blown away by their research findings back then. There are a few theories about the history of sleep and how it's changed over time. The scientific evidence has obviously expanded, and we have different ideas about what sleep does for our bodies. But keep this in mind: there was limited scientific evidence about the underlying function of sleep and why it happened. I think it's important to highlight the timeline to show you how far we've come and the work we have cut out for us.

This won't be an exhaustive list, but a CliffsNotes version of sleep history for the purpose of this book. There are books and articles dedicated to the history and functioning of sleep; I'll add some suggested reading at the end of this book if you'd like to learn more. After reading about the history myself, I've grown to truly appreciate sleep and our lovely scientists who dedicate their lives to answering our burning questions. Let's start with a topic that was trendy back then, before our technological advances, and still is: dreams.

Dreams Were Trending Back Then (and Still Are)

From early on until 1952, researchers strongly focused on dream interpretation and "passive process theory," which, to be honest, makes sleep sound super boring and doesn't give sleep enough credit. Passive process theory suggests that our brains turn off completely and go into a relatively inactive state, and there was limited observation by researchers about our sleep overnight.[6] They didn't have access to polysomnography (a fancy word for a sleep study) back then, and the underlying reason for sleep was relatively unknown. In 1929, Hans Berger discovered different brain waves were observed in humans during their awakened and sleep states, but he still designated sleep as a passive state. I think researchers probably didn't understand the gravity of how important sleep was because they had limited information about it. If it's a passive state and nothing happens, why research it, right?

Wrong. A turn of events generated some interest in sleep in 1953 with the discovery of rapid eye movement (REM) and its association with dreams.[7] Fuck yeah, people were interested in what happens when we sleep! Researchers were captivated by the idea of dreaming states. I kind of think about dreams as somewhat of a parallel life process. You can do anything in your dreams and there are no rules. So, you might not have any poor consequences after waking up, unless it was a nightmare and you were scared. So, if someone bullied you, you could essentially take them to court to get retribution, put peanut butter on all of their door handles, and then wake up like nothing happened. Maybe you dreamt that your bully went to jail for something. Pretty cool. Not saying this has happened in my dreams or anything...

---

6   Dement, W. C. (1998). The study of human sleep: a historical perspective. *Thorax, 53*(3), S2-S7.

7   Aserinsky, E., and Kleitman, N. (1953). Regularly occurring periods of eye motility, and concomitant phenomena, during sleep. *Science, 118*(3062), 273-274.

After World War II, brain waves were recorded overnight at the laboratory of Nathaniel Kleitman at the University of Chicago.[8] The stages of sleep and sleep architecture were studied[9] and gained heightened interest in 1960 with a study about REM deprivation that allowed us to see that dreams may be more likely to be remembered during REM sleep.[10] This captured lots of attention because, at the time, people were captivated by the concept of dreaming and what it all means. And if people are looking to analyze what dreams mean and wonder why humans behave the way they do, they must be interested in psychology.

Think about it, this (after WWII) was around the same time that Freud was becoming popular for his work on dreams as it relates to our unconscious processes.[11] His book *Interpretation of Dreams*[12] was gaining traction and people were interested in dreams. Sleep and early psychology aligned in some way, and as we know, he was the founder of psychoanalysis and influenced modern psychology and psychiatry.

Psychoanalytic psychologists are fascinated with how unconscious and conscious elements of the brain interact to uncover repressed fears or motives. One of Freud's theories suggested that dreams allow us to express ourselves in ways that we may not be able to in our waking life. So, if we wanted to do something wild that was incredibly unacceptable or illegal, well, we can dream about it instead. We might not be conscious of this in our awakened state; our dreams will tell us everything we need to know. Freud's discoveries influenced the field of psychology, but there was way more in store for the sleep world.

---

8   Dement, W., and Kleitman, N. (1957) Cyclic variations in EEG during sleep and their relation to eye movements, body motility, and dreaming. *Electroencephalography and Clinical Neurophysiology*, 9(4), 673-690.

9   Dement, W., and Wolpert, E. (1958). The relation of eye movements, body motility, and external stimuli to dream content. *Journal of Experimental Psychology*, 55(6), 543-553.

10 Dement, W. (1960). The depth of sleep and dream deprivation. *Science, 132*, 1420-1422.

11 See footnote 6.

12 Freud, S. (1900). *The interpretation of dreams*. The Macmillan Company.

Dreams Are Cool, but There's More to It

Over time, sleep became more of a research inquiry rather than a vague, illusive experience that we all shared and never questioned. Have you ever heard of a sleep study? Well, researchers discovered polysomnography (sleep study), which we know today as a sleep study used to diagnose certain sleep disorders, such as sleep apnea. This tool records oxygen levels, blood pressure, brain waves, heart rate, and body movements overnight.[13] It uses electromyography (EMG), electroencephalography (EEG), and electrooculography (EOG) information but most of the time people go to a sleep lab to undergo this study, so they aren't nearly as comfortable because their home and the lab look and feel different.[14]

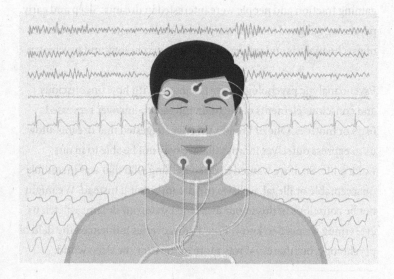

---

13   Rundo, J. V., and Downey III, R. (2019). Chapter 25 - Polysomnography. *Handbook of Clinical Neurology, 160,* 381-392.

14   Portier, F., Portmann, A., Czernichow, P., Vascaut, L., Devin, E., Benhamou, D., Cuvelier, A., And Muir, J. F. (2000). Evaluation of home versus laboratory polysomnography in the diagnosis of sleep apnea syndrome. *American Journal of Respiratory and Critical Care Medicine, 162,* 814-818.

The EOG measures eye movements, the EEG measures brain wave activity, and the EMG measures muscle movements.[15] It was the first tool that provided us with a view into what happens to our brains while we sleep. Later we will chat about the different brain waves and what happens in certain stages of sleep, but this was crucial for the sleep research industry. We know that there are noticeable changes in muscle tone, eye movements, and brain activity during certain sleep stages, and a polysomnography provides an inside view into someone's sleep architecture. We can tell what stage of sleep someone's in, if they're getting enough oxygen overnight, if they're exhibiting any parasomnias (a.k.a. odd behaviors that happen when we sleep) by using a polysomnography. I sometimes think about what it's like to undergo a test like this. You have all these wires attached to stickers that they place on your body to record stuff. Really think about this. Stickers and wires can give us insight into our brains. Holy fuck.

Anyway, if you think of any sort of sleep tracker nowadays, they can mostly detect motion, heart rate, and maybe the time you get into bed, but they aren't entirely accurate or reliable in recording brain waves/activity, blood pressure, or oxygen levels because their intended purpose is different than a medical test. These trackers are helpful, of course, but they aren't as intense as polysomnography and are used for different reasons. Trackers are helpful to instill habits and keeping track of behaviors as it relates to sleep. Maybe it gives you insight into your bed window (a.k.a. the time you got into bed and the time you left your bed) but it might not catch the times you fall asleep or wake up. This is still useful, though. If we compare these trackers to the gold standard (polysomnography), they aren't as accurate (or clinically indicated) for detecting sleep disorders,[16] but these trackers aren't

15   Johns Hopkins Medicine. (2021, Aug. 8). *Sleep study*. https://www.hopkinsmedicine.org/health/treatment-tests-and-therapies/sleep-study.

16   Ameen, M. S., Cheung, L. M., Hauser, T., Hahn, M. A., and Schabus, M. (2019). About the accuracy and problems of consumer devices in the assessment of sleep. *Sensors, 19*(19), 4160.

intended for diagnostic purposes. They are helpful and have shown to be useful for looking at time in bed and some sleep habits,[17] even if they don't give as much accurate information about our sleep architecture as a polysomnography would.

We are advancing quickly as a society, so I'm sure these sleep trackers will become more advanced and accurate because not everyone with a suspected sleep disorder needs polysomnography. For example, this test isn't necessary for diagnosing chronic or acute insomnia, but it is super helpful for sleep apnea. However! There are over seventy sleep disorders, so it's crucial to see a professional for your sleep concerns because each treatment looks different. Regardless, I mostly suggest that my clients fill out a sleep diary,[18] in conjunction with using a tracker application. The sleep diary yields extremely useful data about sleep as it relates to insomnia and behavioral sleep patterns, and it helps us adjust our treatment recommendations (e.g., bed windows, wake times) throughout the CBT-I process. Sheesh, there's so much sleep information out there I have to get back on track with our sleep history lesson.

In November 1972, William Dement (a.k.a. sleep daddy), the leading authority figure on sleep, sleep deprivation, and the diagnosis and treatment of sleep disorders, was determined to make a difference in the sleep world. He and a few sleep researchers banned together and created the first organized sleep medicine course at Stanford University, which still exists today and is known as the Stanford Sleep Disorders Clinic and Research Center.[19] Can you imagine how

---

17   Bhat, S., Ferraris, A., Gupta, D., Mozafarian, M., DeBari, V. A., Gushway-Henry, N., Gowda, S. P., Polos, P. G., Rubinstein, M., Huzaifa, S., and Chokroverty, S. (2015). Is there a clinical role for smartphone sleep apps? Comparison of sleep cycle detection by a smartphone application to polysomnography. *Journal of Clinical Sleep Medicine, 11*(7), 709–715.

18   Maich, K. H. G., Lachowski, A. M., and Carney, C. E. (2018). Psychometric properties of the consensus sleep diary in those with insomnia disorder. *Behavioral Sleep Medicine, 16*(2), 117–134.

19   Stanford Medicine News Center. (2003, Mar. 10). *Stanford sleep research legend Dement teaches his final class.* https://med.stanford.edu/news/all-news/2003/03/stanford-sleep-research-legend-dement-teaches-his-final-class.

difficult researching and studying sleep may have been back then? The researchers leading this program were like, "Hey guys, we have to focus on the thing that nobody knows about, which is sleep, so let's organize a group and figure it out." How vulnerable this must have been, and I'm sure they got some backlash for it. It's never easy starting something from the ground up with limited information and resources to teach others about their findings. Stanford created the first fellowship program accredited by the American Sleep Disorders Association (ASDA), which focuses on training doctors on topics like insomnia, narcolepsy, medications relating to sleep, and sleep surgeries, to name a few.[20] People who graduate from this program are crucial to helping us continue to understand and evaluate sleep disorders and sleep health. I view them as sleep research heroes.

We didn't know many things about sleep, but people complained they were tired and fatigued throughout the day. Dr. Mary Carskadon, professor in the Department of Psychiatry and Human Behavior at the Warren Alpert Medical School of Brown University and one of the most prominent sleep researchers (a.k.a. a sleep queen), decided to learn more about this to help others struggling with sleep issues. She and her colleagues researched the factors that contributed to daytime sleepiness and fatigue, which helped create the Multiple Sleep Latency Test (MSLT),[21] a test that measures these factors. This was important to figure out why people felt sleepy during the day, something most of us still experience. It helps with diagnosing certain disorders. And, shit, who doesn't want to know the reason for their daytime fatigue? Then, there was a huge highlight for sleep research that changed how we view sleep disorders.

20   Stanford Medicine, Division of Sleep Medicine. (n.d.). *Stanford University ACGME sleep medicine fellowship training*. https://med.stanford.edu/sleepdivision/education/sleepmedfellowship.html.

21   Stanford Medicine Health Care. (n.d.). *Multiple sleep latency test (MSLT)*. https://stanfordhealthcare.org/medical-conditions/sleep/narcolepsy/diagnosis/multiple-sleep-latency-test.html.

In 1976, researchers figured out how to treat obstructive sleep apnea (OSA),[22] a medical condition that causes a person to experience apneas during the night, which are episodes of non-breathing. Scary, right? Yes, and important to study because without breathing, well, there's no oxygen to the brain. When there's no oxygen to the brain, that's not good for cardiovascular or brain health. We already knew how to diagnose OSA with polysomnography, but treating it was another story. Researchers were probably like, "Damn, we got all these people out here with episodes of non-breathing overnight and we can't fix it." That must have been such a helpless feeling. Buckle up, though—this story ends on a high note!

In 1980, researchers introduced the continuous positive airway pressure (CPAP) shared by Colin Sullivan to help with obstructive sleep apnea.[23] How fuckin' cool! I mean, talk about leveling up. It was probably one of the most important discoveries for the sleep world in terms of diagnosing sleep disorders and is something we still use today. Eliot Philipson started the research in 1970, but it wasn't fully adopted until June 1980.

OSA is a condition that causes pauses in airflow to the brain because of a blockage in the airway. *Obstructive* means there's something in the way and *apnea* means cessation of breathing, and this all happens while the person is sleeping. You might not even be conscious of it. The CPAP machine works by pushing continuous airflow into the lungs to avoid the apnea episodes from happening altogether.[24] I've seen clients who have more than sixty apneas per night, which means that they technically stopped breathing sixty times! We know

---

22   Guilleminault, C., Tilkian, A., Dement, W. C. (1976) The sleep apnea syndromes. *Annual Review of Medicine, 27*, 465–484.

23   Sullivan, C. E., Berthon-Jones, M., Issa, F.G., and Evans, L. (1981). Reversal of obstructive sleep apnea by continuous positive airway pressure applied through the nares. *The Lancet, 317*(8225), 862–865.

24   Healthline. (2020, Aug. 18). *What is a CPAP machine, and how does it work?* https://www.healthline.com/health/what-is-a-cpap-machine.

that lack of oxygen to the brain is detrimental to our health, and it can cause more issues as we age if this happens for long periods of time. As you can see, this CPAP machine was a great discovery. It can be uncomfortable to sleep with initially. I've helped people with CPAP adherence in therapy and we've worked through these barriers together. Oxygen is more important than comfort, but sometimes it's hard to get to sleep when uncomfortable.

What if there was a permanent solution for sleep apnea that didn't require a big machine? In 1981, Dr. Shiro Fujita shared the Uvulopalatopharyngoplasty (UPPP) with United States researchers, a surgery intended to help with disordered breathing. The procedure removes parts of tissue within the throat to aid airflow.[25] It was a great invention until some patients realized they didn't want to go through a surgical procedure. It was first introduced in 1964 to assist with snoring, but it didn't gain much traction until the 1980s.[26] We've seen the CPAP machine to be effective, so the risks of the UPPP outweigh the benefits. Either way, these researchers and scientists are so badass. They see a problem and try to create a solution for it. Eternally grateful for these folks.

The Inception of Insomnia Treatments

What about psychologists? Throughout all these other research wins, Professor Thomas Borkove started conducting CBT-I studies because this is now the first-line treatment for chronic insomnia, per the American College of Physicians (ACP). It's evolved over the years since its inception.

---

25   Fujita, S., Conway, W., Zorick, F., and Roth, T. (1981). Surgical correction of anatomic abnormalities in obstructive sleep apnea syndrome: uvulopalatopharyngoplasty. *Otolaryngology–Head and Neck Surgery, 89*(6), 923-934.

26   Yaremchuk, K., and Garcia-Rodriguez, L. (2017). The history of sleep surgery. *Advances in Oto-Rhino-Laryngology, 80,* 17-21. https://www.karger.com/Article/Pdf/470683.

What about behavioral interventions, like sleep hygiene? These
interventions for insomnia, such as CBT-I, weren't created in one
shot. Researchers weren't like, "Let's sit down and create this protocol
all at once." They pulled from various other interventions. CBT-I
is an accumulation of several interventions, which makes it super
dynamic. Before the '70s, relaxation strategies were the main modality
for treating insomnia, such as deep, diaphragmatic breathing and
progressive muscle relaxation strategies. These techniques are helpful
for insomnia when used separately, but we've seen that they are the
most effective when used all together, including a few below.

In the 1970s, Richard Bootzin developed stimulus control therapy,
which helps us mentally associate the bed with sleepiness[27] and
is arguably one of the most important components of insomnia
treatment. There were a few discoveries throughout the years that
helped shape CBT-I. In the late 1970s, psychologist Peter Haur
introduced sleep hygiene, basic behavioral strategies to enhance
sleep.[28] It's mostly the stuff you hear about—keeping the bedroom
cool and dark, limiting caffeine and napping, and exercising so that
you can fall asleep soundly. Additionally, in the 1980s, Dr. Spielman
and his colleagues developed sleep restriction therapy,[29] which limits
bed lounging and increases the time in bed that someone sleeps. He
also suggested there is no single cause for insomnia, but includes
predisposing, precipitating, and perpetuating factors,[30] which we
touched on in Chapter 1.

---

27   Bootzin, R.R. (1972). Stimulus control treatment for insomnia. *Proceedings of the 80th Annual
     American Psychological Association Convention,* 395-396.

28   Hauri, P. (1977). *Current concepts: The sleep disorders.* Upjohn.

29   See footnote 1.

30   See footnote 1.

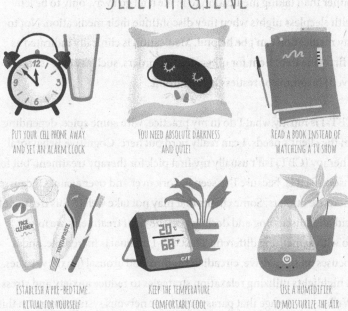

SLEEP HYGIENE

PUT YOUR CELL PHONE AWAY AND SET AN ALARM CLOCK

YOU NEED ABSOLUTE DARKNESS AND QUIET

READ A BOOK INSTEAD OF WATCHING A TV SHOW

ESTABLISH A PRE-BEDTIME RITUAL FOR YOURSELF

KEEP THE TEMPERATURE COMFORTABLY COOL

USE A HUMIDIFIER TO MOISTURIZE THE AIR

Three separate columns: stimulus control therapy, sleep hygiene, and sleep restriction. I can provide more info for each if that's helpful]

If I can give you a quick hint, all of these interventions are included in the traditional CBT-I framework that we still use today. From the 1990s and into the 2000s, CBT-I was formulated into a framework that has been validated and thoroughly researched for those with insomnia. Over time, CBT-I has become the first-line treatment for chronic insomnia, even over psychotropic medications,[31] and still is the most helpful intervention for this type of insomnia. This was a huge step for psychologists and other therapists who assist their clients

31   O'Brien, E. M., and Boland, E. M. (2020). CBT-I is an efficacious, first-line treatment for insomnia: Where we need to go from here. A commentary on the application of Tolin's criteria to cognitive behavioral therapy for insomnia. *Clinical Psychology: Science and Practice, 27*(4).

with sleep issues because people can take time to work on themselves rather than taking medication to make it all go away, only to be left with sleepless nights when they discontinue their medication. Not to say medication can't be helpful. Medication is clinically indicated as a first-line treatment for other sleep disorders, such as acute (short-lived) insomnia or restless leg syndrome.

CBT-I is mostly what I do in my practice, with some spice, depending on the client's needs. I can really nerd out here. Cognitive Behavioral Therapy (CBT) isn't usually my first pick for therapy treatment, but for insomnia it is, because I've seen it work over and over again. Of course, there are outliers. Some clients that may not take well to this treatment, and after discussing and deciding on the right treatment, we might go with something different. The CBT-I manual is incredible, and it focuses on sleep drive, circadian rhythm, and arousal (anxiety) issues. It highlights utilizing relaxation strategies to reduce anxiety and stress. We have to engage that parasympathetic nervous system (more on this later)! It focuses on what we can control rather than saying, "Here's a pill; come back in a few months." Medication is helpful but not in this way. We want people to feel empowered, even if while taking sleep medications. I also like to be mindful of the client's culture, race, language, ability level, and gender, just to name a few, because every person needs something different.

Sleep Research Becomes Even More Important

Let's fast forward to the 1990s, when researchers studied the impact of disordered breathing during sleep and deprivation on cardiovascular health, which was monumental.[32] The American Sleep Disorders

---

32   See footnote 6.

Association was created, and sleep health was finally recognized as something to be included in healthcare and health-related research. Fuck yeah! At the time, Obstructive Sleep Apnea (OSA) affected about thirty million people, and these researchers were bringing to light a medical issue that was crucial to human health and well-being. Most notably, The National Commission on Sleep Disorders Research highlighted that sleep education was severely lacking in the medical curriculum[33] in American schools. It all starts with awareness, and look at us now.

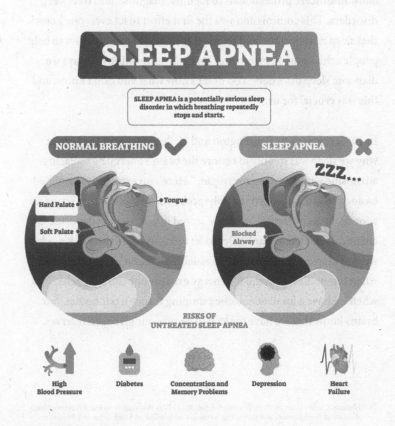

SLEEP APNEA

SLEEP APNEA is a potentially serious sleep disorder in which breathing repeatedly stops and starts.

NORMAL BREATHING ✓

Hard Palate
Soft Palate
Tongue

SLEEP APNEA ✗

ZZZ...

Blocked Airway

RISKS OF
UNTREATED SLEEP APNEA

High Blood Pressure

Diabetes

Concentration and Memory Problems

Depression

Heart Failure

33   Rosen, R. C., Rosekind, M., Rosevear, C., Cole, W. E., and Dement, W. C. (1993). Physician education in sleep and sleep disorders: a national survey of US medical schools. *Sleep*, *16*(3), 249-254.

In 1993, The National Commission on Sleep Disorders Research published an executive summary called *Wake Up America! A National Sleep Alert Executive Summary*,[34] which highlighted key recommendations to help spread awareness about sleep health and how to engage in the early detection of sleep disorders. The commission suggested several areas of growth, one being to cultivate an environment of scientific understanding about sleep and sleep-related disorders and to provide this information to the public. This would help the public be more informed about sleep wellness and allow healthcare professionals to identify, diagnose, and treat sleep disorders. This commission was the first effort to let everyone know that sleep is important, and we must continue to explore ways to help people achieve quality sleep and continue innovating the ways we diagnose sleep disorders. You don't know what you don't know, and this was crucial for us.

In 1995, researchers Bennington and Heller noted that the reason why we sleep was mainly to restore the brain's energy by replacing adenosine with glycogen overnight.[35] Here's an extremely simplified biology lesson: Glycogen is a polysaccharide of glucose that serves as a form of energy storage, which is stored in our brain. Adenosine is a chemical released in our bodies to let us know we're tired (a.k.a. when we don't have any more readily available glycogen). It gets released when our bodies' demand for energy exceeds our cell's capacity.[36] So, when we have a lot of adenosine pumping through our bodies, our brains know that we have to sleep to restore our glycogen reserves.

34 National Commission on Sleep Disorders Research. (1993). *Wake up America. A National Sleep Alert executive summary. A report of the National Commission on Sleep Disorders Research.*

35 Benington, J. H., and Heller, C. H. (1995). Restoration of brain energy metabolism as the function of sleep. *Progress in Neurobiology, 45*(4), 347–360.

36 Stanford News. (1996, Jan. 16). *Stanford researchers suggest how sleep re-charges the brain.* https://news.stanford.edu/pr/96/960116sleep.html.

This was a big discovery because adenosine is something that we still highlight today in insomnia treatment. In 2001, Joshua Gooley and a few researchers found that certain cells in the retina (within our eyes) communicate with the brain's circadian clock to inform it of receiving light or dark information.[37] If we expose ourselves to light before bed it suppresses melatonin secretion (yikes—melatonin helps with our sleep cycles). In 2003, Eugen Tarnow posed a long-term memory excitation theory about dreams, suggesting that dreams and memories are connected and that dreams are the brain's way of processing long-term memories.[38] It was similar to Freud's theory on dreams.

This isn't an exhaustive list of the historical literature, but food for thought as we think about how far we've come within the sleep health world. We've made some pretty amazing discoveries and there is still a lot that we don't know about sleep. Most of our research about sleep is relatively new, too. Of course, some older theories have been tested and retested for validity and reliability. Okay, I know what you're thinking: "I get the history; now what?" Well, it's good that you're here because if you waited for everything to be discovered, well, that might happen long after you've passed away. So, better to get in now when we are still discovering stuff about sleep! But before we move on, what the hell *is* sleep? We know there's a need for it, but what does it do for us?

---

37   Gooley, J. J., Chamberlain, K., Smith, K. A., Khalsa, S. B. S., Rajaratnam, S. M. W., Van Reen, E., Zeitzer, J. M., Czeisler, C. A., and Lockley, S. W. (2011). Exposure to room light before bedtime suppresses melatonin onset and shortens melatonin duration in humans. *The Journal of Clinical Endocrinology and Metabolism, 96*(3), E463-E472.

38   Tarnow, E. (2003). How dreams and memory may be related. *Neuropsychoanalysis, 5*(2), 177-182.

What Even Is Sleep? (The Basics)

I can't convince you to care about your ZZZs without chatting about the amazing underpinnings of sleep. It's too intriguing not to talk about here. We can go into a vortex thinking and talking about sleep, so I'm going to touch on the important concepts but know that there is way more to sleep than even what I can write in this book.

There are a few different definitions of sleep. Researchers Zielinski, McKenna, and McCarley (2016) define sleep as "reduced body movement and electromyographic activity, reduced responsiveness to external stimuli, closed eyes, reduced breathing rates, and altered body position and brain wave architecture."[39] The Merriam-Webster dictionary states that sleep is, "the natural, easily reversible periodic state of many living things that is marked by the absence of wakefulness and by the loss of consciousness of one's surroundings, is accompanied by a typical body posture (such as lying down with the eyes closed), the occurrence of dreaming, and changes in brain activity and physiological functioning, is made up of cycles of non-REM sleep and REM sleep, and is usually considered essential to the restoration and recovery of vital bodily and mental functions."[40] Sounds pretty fricken serious.

Basically, sleep is an involuntary process that helps us regain some juice for certain functions so that we can keep doing the damn thing (the damn thing = living). I'm sure you can envision what this looks

---

39   Zielinski, M. R., McKenna, J. T., and McCarley, R. W. (2016). Functions and mechanisms of sleep. *AIMS Neuroscience, 3*(1), 67-104.

40   Merriam-Webster. (n.d.). *Sleep definition & meaning.* https://www.merriam-webster.com/dictionary/sleep.

and feels like because we all do it. Maybe we sleep differently than this, but it's a shared experience among most species. Most of us view the concept of sleep as drifting off into the unconscious abyss and waking up a few hours later feeling either more tired than we did going to sleep or way more rested. We might have a few dreams here and there, but overall it's a pretty regular process for most of us. (Of course, everyone sleeps differently, and sleep might be a point of contention for some. It might feel unsafe or remind us of past experiences that cause anxiety or depression.)

We rely on polysomnographic data to understand the changes that happen during sleep compared to our awakened state, which is the presence of certain brain waves.[41] These brain waves are indications of different stages of sleep. We'll talk about these waves later (surf's up).

The concept of sleep has evolved since we've been able to learn more about it. We have more information about its purposes and how it can help us. On average, we spend about a third of our lives sleeping.[42] It seems like a pretty big deal if we need so much of it. There are also steep costs for not sleeping well or experiencing issues with our sleep. It affects our daytime functioning and may affect us on a cellular level. We don't see this or feel it directly, but we might have other symptoms that let us know our cells aren't functioning properly due to lack of sleep.

I remember reading a study from 2004 that gave me a view into what lack of sleep does for us as a society. At the time, researchers estimated the annual cost of insomnia at almost 100 billion dollars, which might include costs for doctor's visits, accidents, alcohol consumption, or

---

41   See footnote 39.

42   Wurr, M. (n.d.). *Notes & queries: The body beautiful*. The Guardian. https://www.theguardian.com/notesandqueries/query/0,5753,-50504,00.html.

medications.[43] I can only imagine how much it is now. Well, in 2017 it was pretty much the same, about 100 billion per year.[44] I can't even imagine a million dollars, let alone a billion. Regardless of how much it costs us financially, it truly impacts the quality of our lives. For example, a lack of quality sleep may pose health-related consequences, such as diabetes, cancer, and cardiovascular issues.[45] Big yikes!

Although we've made some great strides in knowing more about sleep, researchers are still investigating the underpinnings of sleep. We know we need it; we need a certain amount of it, depending on our age, and we also need quality sleep. Ever thought about having one quality friend rather than several acquaintances? It's kind of like that. We want to nurture our relationship have with our sleep and focus more on the quality of the experience rather than the quantity, no matter how many hours or to say we slept for "x" hours. We'll chat more about this in a bit.

The idea of sleep has changed over time, too. I'd imagine our bodies have had to adjust since the invention of electricity, shift work, social media, and televisions (we'll talk later about how exposure to light affects our sleep-wake cycles). We are more stressed than ever because we are focused not only on survival but thriving, and we know that stress and anxiety affect our sleep health. We are facing a lot of challenges as a society, such as adjusting our societal norms, trying to make life more inclusive for all people, and still fighting an uphill battle for certain marginalized populations. I'm not sure we dealt with the same societal issues back then; I'm sure our stressors looked different, or they were less discussed, at least. Most of us are "waking

---

43   Morin, C. M. (2004). Cognitive-behavioral approaches to the treatment of insomnia. *Journal of Clinical Psychiatry, 65*(Suppl. 16), 33–40.

44   Wickwire, E. M., Shaya, F. T., and Scharf, S. M. (2016). Health economics of insomnia treatments: The return on investment for a good night's sleep. *Sleep Medicine Reviews, 30,* 72–82.

45   See footnote 4.

up" in different ways, and I'd imagine one of these ways includes how sleep affects our functioning.

Function of Sleep

What we do know is that we don't know everything about sleep. Kinda weird, right? We have a puzzle with a few missing pieces and nobody knows where to find them. Well, sleep researchers are on the hunt for them, thankfully! We've come a long way, as we've seen from history, but there's still so much to uncover about sleep. Researchers suggest a few reasons why we sleep, and they are still investigating the idea of sleep in general. So, just know that sleep is a basic human need that we still need more information about.

Sometimes we get hooked on the idea of "I need eight hours of sleep." I know I did for a while. But what's more important is getting quality sleep to ensure that our bodies can function the next day and overnight. The numbers matter, but quality matters more. Imagine intentionally working on a project for six hours versus haphazardly working on that same project for ten hours. The outcome may be different. Even if the outcome is the same, we were more intentional with our time. With six hours, we feel less frustration about spending so much more time on a project to get the same result. Our relationship with quality sleep is kinda like this.

There's a *lot* that happens overnight. It's almost like we're the head supervisor and our bodies are having a long meeting that we're not invited to. We don't know what goes on in that meeting overnight, but we know it's essential for our bodies to function properly the next day. We can assume that one function of sleep is energy restoration[46]

---

46   See footnote 35.

and autonomic nervous system functioning[47] because we know what it physically feels like if we aren't sleeping well. We're exhausted, we can't think straight, and it's difficult to get anything done or communicate effectively.

Hidden Gems for Our Functioning: Involuntary Biological Processes

I know the term *autonomic nervous system* sounds fancy. Well, it is pretty fabulous (and essential). It regulates involuntary processes (a.k.a. the processes that seem automatic that we don't have to consciously control)—breathing, digestion, heart rate, or sexual arousal.[48] Of course, people have issues with these functions. Our autonomic nervous system is divided into three parts: sympathetic, parasympathetic, and enteric. The sympathetic nervous system regulates our stress response (a.k.a. fight-flight-or-freeze response), and the parasympathetic nervous system controls our relaxation response. Sleep helps regulate these processes, which may affect how we deal with stress or our ability to relax. The enteric system controls our gastrointestinal system and is connected to the sympathetic nervous system.

Let's dive in deeper. As we transition from being awake to falling asleep, our sympathetic nervous system (stress response) isn't nearly as loud because we are preparing to be unconscious. To be unconscious, we may assume we have to be somewhat in a relaxed state, which is why the parasympathetic nervous system signals are

---

47   Zoccoli, G., and Amici, R. (2020). Sleep and autonomic nervous system. *Current Opinion in Physiology, 15*, 128–133.

48   Waxenbaum, J. A., Reddy, V., and Varacallo, M. (2021). *Anatomy, autonomic nervous system.* StatPearls Publishing.

louder.[49] In our deeper stages of sleep (e.g., non-REM stage three), our parasympathetic nervous system is dominant, breathing slows down, and our bodies engage in metabolic recovery.[50] This helps us engage in those restorative activities, such as repairing muscles and tissue, mental reorganization, maintaining body temperature, or restoring our bodies' energy reserve. This is quite the opposite of what happens when we are stressed. When stressed, our sympathetic nervous system activates, and we notice more of the stress hormone cortisol. We aren't worried about restoring our bodies' resources because we are worried about survival. So, sleep is important for repairing the things that we do when we're awake. Survival mode isn't helpful when we sleep.

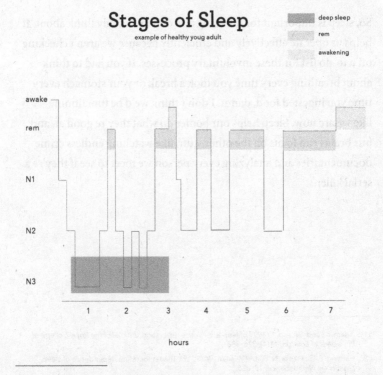

Stages of Sleep
example of healthy youg adult

deep sleep
rem
awakening

---

49 Miglis, M.G. "Sleep and the autonomic nervous system." In *Sleep and neurologic disease*, pp. 227–244. Academic Press, 2017.

50 See footnote 49.

People say, "If you're working out, your body needs rest to repair its muscles." Well, that might also happen while we sleep. Some experts believe one function of sleep is to repair our cells and tissues.[51] Experts also believe sleep helps to maintain our core body temperature, which is important for our sleep-wake cycles. Our bodies experience a drop in core temperature at certain points in our twenty-four-hour cycle, which serves as a cue to prepare for sleep.[52] This happens to animals, too. On the other hand, increasing core temperature lets the body know it's time to stay awake.[53] As you can see, if we can't maintain or regulate our body temperature, it may affect our sleep. We've seen that those with insomnia may have inconsistent body temperature changes that aren't aligned with their preferred bedtime or bed window.[54]

So, sleep is important for the things we don't normally think about. It helps us operate effectively and efficiently because we aren't checking off a to-do list for these involuntary processes. If you had to think about breathing every time you took a break or your stomach every time you ingested food, damn. I don't think we'd be functioning like we are now. Sleep helps our bodies do what they're good at, and our brains can focus on the other stuff, like watching endless crime documentaries and analyzing every person we meet to see if they're a serial killer.

---

51   Adam, K., and Oswald, I. (1977). Sleep is for tissue restoration. *Journal of the Royal College of Physicians of London, 11*(4), 376–388.

52   Harding, E. C., Franks, N. P., and Wisden, W. (2019). The temperature dependence of sleep. *Frontiers in Neuroscience, 13*, 336.

53   Okamoto-Mizuno, K., and Mizuno, K. (2012). Effects of thermal environment on sleep and circadian rhythm. *Journal of Physiological Anthropology, 31*, 14.

54   See footnote 53.

Remembered Gems: Our Memory

Something a little less physical but equally important is our memory. There are so many different types of memory, and quality sleep is essential to acquire and store new information.[55] Some researchers suggest that newly stored memories happen during sleep rather than while we are awake.[56] So, we acquire all of the information in our awakened state, and we sleep it off to store that information as a new memory, also known as memory consolidation. This is one of those things that we don't directly *feel* or have an awareness of, but it's important for us as humans because it would be difficult to function without the concept of memory.

If we think about it even more deeply, we have sensory, working, short-term, and long-term memory. I like to look at this from a stage perspective rather than seeing these as all different. There are a bunch of theories on this, so this isn't the only way researchers see memory. We see or experience something in the environment and engage our senses, we may manipulate that information, then we store it in short-term memory. Some memories get stored long-term for specific reasons. As discussed earlier, this is a simplified view of memory and there are so many more complex parts, which I will be missing here. Researchers write entire books and articles on the concept of our memory; it truly fascinates me.

---

55 Diekelmann, S., and Born, J. (2010). The memory function of sleep. *Nature Reviews Neuroscience*, *11*(2), 114-126.

56 See footnote 55.

Types of Memory

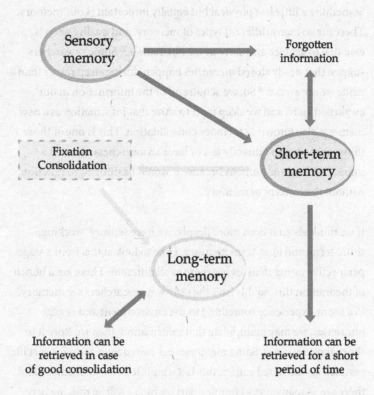

inspired by Figure 4.1.5 Attention on https://scientistcafe.com/notes/
introtopsychology/perception-and-attention.html]

Sensory memory holds information for only about a second or two, such as noises in the environment or tasting a new type of food. It engages our senses, and these may go into short-term or long-term memory. Otherwise, we forget about these experiences pretty quickly. For example, you might not remember a certain sound unless something prompts you to remember it. Isn't this wild?

Short-term memory is our ability to recall or hold information for about thirty seconds,[57] otherwise we lose it and it doesn't become a memory. For example, we may try to remember an address or phone number while we type it into our phone. We don't usually remember this after we've written it down unless there's a specific reason. Working memory is similar to short-term memory but includes our ability to take in information and "work" it into a different form.[58] It's our ability to manipulate information.[59] For example, if you see the numbers 1-2-3-4-5, you'll use working memory to say these numbers backward, 5-4-3-2-1. It's helpful when solving certain problems or using critical thinking skills, too.

And then we have (in my opinion) the main character, long-term memory. I picture long-term memory as a queen with a lot of glitter and demanding presence. Long-term memory is divided into two groups: implicit (unconscious) and explicit (conscious).[60] Implicit memories are memories that influence our behavior, but we aren't consciously aware of them. For example, procedural memory helps us engage in familiar tasks such as riding a bike, walking, or physically picking up items. We don't have to think about doing these things; they almost seem automatic.[61] Explicit memories are those that we are consciously aware of, such as your twenty-fifth birthday party (episodic memory) or facts about the world that you haven't experienced in real time but have knowledge of,[62] such as the fact that

---

57 Jonides, J., Lewis, R. L., Nee, D. E., Lustig, C. A., Berman, M. G., and Moore, K. S. (2008). The mind and brain of short-term memory. *Annual Review of Psychology, 59*, 193-224.

58 Aben, B., Stapert, S., and Blokland, A. (2012). About the distinction between working memory and short-term memory. *Frontiers in Psychology, 3*, 301.

59 Nairne, J. S., & Neath, I. (2013). Sensory and working memory. In A. F. Healy, R. W. Proctor, & I. B. Weiner (Eds.), *Handbook of psychology: Experimental psychology* (pp. 419-445). John Wiley & Sons, Inc.

60 Norris, D. (2017). Short-term memory and long-term memory are still different. *Psychological Bulletin, 143*(9), 992-1009.

61 Queensland Brain Institute. (n.d.). *Types of memory.* https://qbi.uq.edu.au/brain-basics/memory/types-memory.

62 See footnote 61.

dolphins turn off half of their brains when they sleep.[63] You haven't personally experienced this but have read this fact somewhere and can recall it.

Now what does this have to do with sleep? Well, the process where this information becomes encoded and stored occurs during slow-wave and REM sleep.[64] "Okay, Kristen, what does this really mean?" Well, if we are awake to experience life in real time, we don't store this information as a memory during that time. We are creating memories in real time, but it's up to our brains to consolidate this information and know where to put it, which happens during sleep. The hippocampus is crucial for this process,[65] as it acts as a distribution center for information before it's sent to long-term memory, which happens while we sleep. So we can experience all the fun we want in life, but it may not become a memory without sleep.

I was studying for the Examination for Professional Practice in Psychology (EPPP), the long, complex test to become licensed as a clinical psychologist, and I had to study so much for it. I had trouble with the memory section and a professor once asked me, "Do you remember that hippo on campus?" I'm like, "…what campus?" They were like, "Our campus; don't you remember seeing it?" I was so confused. They said, "Well, now you won't forget that the hippocampus is involved in memory processes." So when I'm struggling to prioritize my sleep, I think of a cute little hippo running around holding all of my memories. It helps me think about how important it is to focus on my sleep health for my brain.

---

63 Oleksenko, A. I., Mukhametov, L. M., Polyakova, I. G., Supin, A. Y., and Kovalzon, V. M. (1992). Unihemispheric sleep deprivation in bottlenose dolphins. *Journal of Sleep Research, 1,* 40–44.

64 Born, J., and Wilhelm, I. (2012). System consolidation of memory during sleep. *Psychological Research, 76,* 192–203.

65 See footnote 64.

In my opinion, our memories truly create our life as humans. If you think about it, we experience life and sometimes reflect on the good times, bad times, or neutral times. We remember how people made us feel, or if we experienced fleeting feelings of love or lust. We remember that great trip we took with friends. We also might remember ways that society has failed us, such as the barriers to accessing quality healthcare, or the inability for certain people to live above the poverty line. All of these experiences create who we are, and it's a lens through which we experience our lives in real time. Memory is so important, and this is part of the reason why you should care about your sleep. Life looks different without memories.

And some memories we don't want to remember because they're so traumatic. I get it. Some of them you could do without, right? I think about how our memories shape us and how acknowledging these memories also validates our experiences as humans. If we simply forget about them then it doesn't capture the true essence of our individuality and uniqueness as human beings, although remembering may be painful at times.

Cognition

Do you ever wake up from a shitty night of sleep and think, "Damn, how am I going to get through the day?" Yeah, I've been there. You move slower. You're more irritable. Little things bother you. It's hard to pay attention. You can't wait for the day to be over to lay in bed, and once you do, you might still not be exhausted enough to fall asleep quickly.

When we don't have enough restorative sleep, our brains go into overdrive. Our neurons work too hard to achieve what would normally be (somewhat) effortless after a good night's rest. A poor night of sleep makes our bodies work twice as hard to do the same things they normally do. Work smarter, not harder, right? We might not feel it on a cellular level, but our bodies react to poor-quality sleep in various ways. We might have slower reaction time, make more mistakes at work or home, or have difficulty remembering things.[66]

And the consequences of these experiences can be quite drastic if we get deep. If we constantly struggle with paying attention at work, focusing on the things that are meaningful to us, or struggling to remember or think about things, that truly affects our relationships, work, self-esteem, and overall life fulfillment. The things that we're already dealing with may feel insurmountable, and it's difficult for us to have a sense of esteem to continue plugging through our days. We start to feel sluggish and might spend more time at the doctor's office, calling out of work, or trying to get behind the wheel to drive home after feeling exhausted.

So that silly thing that we call "sleep" can throw off our entire life. And if we do this day after day, week after week, year after year... Well, you know where I'm going with this.

Before we can even have the capacity to create or store memories, we need to be cognitively aware of what's happening around us. Cognition involves a whole host of processes but is mostly known as "thinking." Thinking can also involve perceiving, reasoning, or learning.[67] When we are acutely aware and think about our thoughts, that's called metacognition.[68] It's the critical awareness of thoughts and is mostly involved in learning. You might engage in metacognition in

---

66   Suni, E., and Dimitriu, A. (2022). *Sleep deprivation*. Sleep Foundation. https://www.sleepfoundation.org/sleep-deprivation.

67   Encyclopedia Britannica. (n.d.). *Cognition*. https://www.britannica.com/topic/cognition-thought-process.

68   Livingston, J. A. (2003). *Metacognition: An overview*. https://files.eric.ed.gov/fulltext/ED474273.pdf.

therapy or the critical thinking involved in an academic class. Yeah, we can get pretty deep here, but let's focus on the function of cognition as it relates to sleep.

Cognition is more than thoughts. It includes our ability to pay attention, use our language capabilities, and engage in mental reasoning.[69] Sleep also helps us restore our executive functions, which are mental functions that aid in self-control, decision-making, planning, and memory.[70] We've seen that sleep deprivation can slow down our reaction time,[71] increase continuing patterns of thoughts that aren't super helpful for us (also known as perseveration),[72] and reduce communication skills and creative thinking.[73,74] People who sleep well after learning typically perform better on memory retrieval tests than those who are sleep deprived.[75]

These executive functions noted above are important for us as humans. Executive functions are our higher-order cognitive processes, which include abstract thinking, strategic goal planning, problem-solving, controlling impulses, and self-monitoring.[76] These are mostly regulated by the prefrontal regions of the frontal lobe of our brains, a.k.a. the prefrontal cortex (PFC). The PFC is divided into a few parts: the medial lateral and orbital prefrontal cortex.[77] I like to call this

---

69   Diekelmann, S. (2014). Sleep for cognitive enhancement. *Frontiers in Systems Neuroscience, 8*(46).

70   Tucker, A. M., Whitney, P., Belenky, G., Hinson, J. M., Van Dongen, H. P. A. (2022). Effects of sleep deprivation on dissociated components of executive functioning. *Sleep, 33*(1), 47-57.

71   Van Dongen, H. P. A., Maislin, G., Mullington, J. M., and Dinges, D. F. (2003). The cumulative cost of additional wakefulness: dose-response effects on neurobehavioral functions and sleep physiology from chronic sleep restriction and total sleep deprivation. *Sleep, 26*(2), 117-126.

72   Retey, J.V.; Adam, M.; Gottselig, J., Khatami, R., Dürr, R., Achermann, P., and Landolt, H. (2006). Adenosinergic mechanisms contribute to individual differences in sleep deprivation-induced changes in neurobehavioral function and brain rhythmic activity. *Journal of Neuroscience, 26*(41), 10472-10479.

73   Harrison, Y., and Horne, J. A. (1998). Sleep loss impairs short and novel language tasks having a prefrontal focus. *Journal of Sleep Research, 7*(2), 95-100.

74   See footnote 69.

75   Rasch, B., and Born, J. (2013). About sleep's role in memory. *Physiological Reviews, 93*(2), 681-766.

76   See footnote 70.

77   GoodTherapy. *Prefrontal cortex.* https://www.goodtherapy.org/blog/psychpedia/prefrontal-cortex.

general region the CEO of our brain. This region is the planner and decision maker; it inhibits us from making shitty decisions and helps us plan our day. So you can only imagine what happens to this part of the brain when we aren't sleeping well.

So, I know what you might be thinking. "Kristen, will a *ton* of sleep enhance my cognitive performance beyond the healthy limits?" Not necessarily. Sleep helps restore cognition to a normal human function; it doesn't enhance cognition beyond this.[78] But, sleep can help us grow in general.

Growth and Development

A few people in my life have kids, and I thought, *Damn, babies sleep so much!* Yeah, there's a reason for that. The National Sleep Foundation suggests that, on average, healthy newborns need about fourteen to seventeen hours of sleep per night, and infants need about twelve to sixteen hours per night, which is drastically different from healthy adults, which is (on average) around seven to nine hours of sleep.[79, 80] Adults are fully grown, newborn and infants aren't, which means they need sleep to aid in their growth and development.[81] Growth hormone is secreted overnight from the anterior pituitary gland, and you guessed it, this helps us grow.[82] So, yeah, babies grow while they sleep; isn't this amazing?

---

78   Sandberg, A. (2011). Cognition enhancement: upgrading the brain. In J. Savulescu, R. ter Muelen, and G. Kahane (Eds.), *Enhancing Human Capacities* (pp. 71–91). Wiley-Blackwell.

79   Camerota, M., Tully, K. P., Grimes, M., Gueron-Sela, N., and Propper, C. b. (2018). Assessment of infant sleep: How well do multiple methods compare? *Sleep, 41*(10), zsy146.

80   See footnote 77.

81   Dereymaeker, A., Pillay, K., Vervisch, J., DeVos, M., Van Huffel, S., Jansen, K., and Naulaers, G. (2017). Review of sleep-EEG in preterm and term neonates. *Early Human Development, 113,* 87–103.

82   Chokroverty, S. (1994). An overview of sleep. *Sleep Disorders Medicine,* 7–16.

Even as young children and adolescents, we don't need as much sleep as when we were newborns or infants, but we still need more sleep than adults. The National Sleep Foundation suggests that teenagers need about eight to ten hours of sleep.[83] I can't tell you how many people have said to me, "I wish I could sleep as much as I did in high school. I remember sleeping through the night and just feeling overall rested." Well, same. We might not remember the poor nights of sleep we had, and there's also another reason for this.

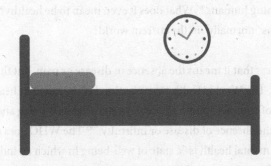

HOW MUCH SLEEP DO WE REALLY NEED ?

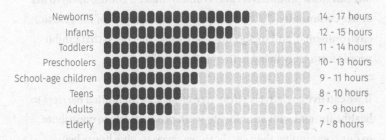

Newborns	14 - 17 hours
Infants	12 - 15 hours
Toddlers	11 - 14 hours
Preschoolers	10 - 13 hours
School-age children	9 - 11 hours
Teens	8 - 10 hours
Adults	7 - 9 hours
Elderly	7 - 8 hours

Our bodies were concerned with different things during childhood and adolescence. We were focused on growth and coming out of

83 Hirshkowitz, M., Whiton, K., Albert, S. M., Alessi, C. Bruni, O., DonCarlos, L., Hazen, N., Herman, J., Katz, E. S., Kheirandish-Gozal, L., Neubauer, D. N., O'Donnell, A. E., Ohayon, M., Peever, J., Rawding, R., Sachdeva, R. C., Setters, B., Vitiello, M. V., … and Adams, P. J. (2015). National Sleep Foundation's sleep time duration recommendations: methodology and results summary. *Sleep Health 1*(1), 40-43.

puberty, and our brains were technically still forming. On top of it, we may have been focused on things other than sleep, such as making friends or learning what kinds of people we were attracted to, or if our caregivers would come home that day. In my opinion, we are way more focused on sleep as we age. Ask any kid if they care about sleep. They might tell you they want to do fun stuff rather than sleep.

Probably one of the most important factors to consider, in my humble opinion, is that these sleep recommendations are based on healthy functioning humans.[84] What does it even mean to be healthy? Who functions "normally" in the current world?

I can guess that it means the absence of disease or pain, but that's not the case. The World Health Organization (WHO) defines health as "a state of complete physical, mental and social well-being and not merely the absence of disease or infirmity."[85] The WHO goes on to say that mental health is "a state of well-being in which an individual realizes his or her own abilities, can cope with the normal stresses of life, can work productively and is able to make a contribution to his or her community."[86] I can't help but think about all of the genetic, environmental, and socioeconomic factors (barriers) that inhibit people from truly living to their full potential.

If we can live a relatively stress-free lifestyle, with limited barriers to healthcare, and with an ability to work productively to contribute to our community, then yes, I can see seven to nine hours being achievable for healthy adults. However, that's not the case for most of us. How can we live up to a standard like this when most of us have stress that is out of our control?

---

84   Suni, E., and Singh, A. (2022). *How much sleep do we really need?* Sleep Foundation, https://www.sleepfoundation.org/how-sleep-works/how-much-sleep-do-we-really-need.

85   World Health Organization. (2022, June). *Mental health: Strengthening our response.* https://www.who.int/news-room/fact-sheets/detail/mental-health-strengthening-our-response.

86   See footnote 85.

Sleep Architecture

Now that we have a rough idea of why sleep is important for our
health, let's talk about the structure of sleep. Quality sleep and sleep
architecture are equally important to the actual number of hours
of sleep, although we know these numbers are averages for healthy
functioning. For example, you can technically experience ten hours
of sleep with multiple awakenings and you might wake up feeling
unrested. However, if you sleep seven hours with only two awakenings
(about two awakenings are normal for healthy functioning adults),
your brain has a higher likelihood of obtaining the number of sleep
cycles needed to restore functioning. Okay, but what are sleep cycles,
and why are they important? Glad you asked :)

Non-REM vs. REM

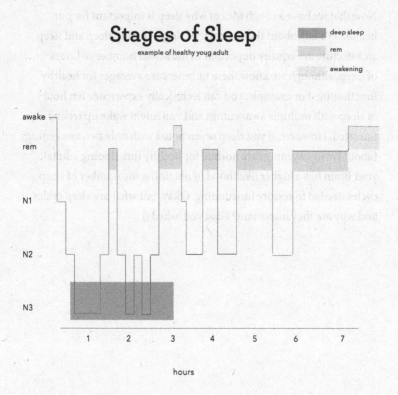

So, if we're discussing the topic of "what even is sleep?" we should cover non-REM. There are two different types of sleep: REM (rapid eye movement sleep) and non-REM (non-rapid eye movement sleep).[87]

So, we have three stages of non-REM sleep (N1, N2, and N3), which are technically different from REM sleep. N1, our lightest non-REM stage, lasts on average between five and ten minutes, and you can be

---

87   Cleveland Clinic. (2020). *Sleep basics*. https://my.clevelandclinic.org/health/articles/12148-sleep-basics.

woken up pretty easily in this stage. It's basically your body dozing off. As you're falling asleep, you'll notice hypnic jerks, a.k.a. quick muscle jerking motions, which happen to most of us as we are in this stage. They are nothing to be concerned about and give us an idea that our bodies are potentially getting ready to go into deeper stages of sleep.[88]

Then we drift into N2, which lasts about ten to thirty minutes, where we experience a drop in core body temperature and eye movement ceases.[89] Sounds scary as hell, but our brain is slowing down to prepare for the deepest stage of sleep, N3. Of course, some of us spend more or less time in each sleep stage, and sometimes these differences are drastic based on medical concerns, medication, or other bodily experiences.

The deepest stage of sleep is N3. We all long for "deep sleep," but in my opinion, efficient sleep architecture is more important than one single stage of sleep. We want to flow through all stages so that our bodies get what they need. People who don't obtain enough sleep from all the stages may experience issues with emotions and physical health,[90] which are what makes us human. Anyway, we can detect deep sleep by the presence of delta brain waves, and we spend most of our time in deep sleep toward the first half of the night. Then, the latter end of the night consists of REM sleep. Deep sleep helps with our creativity[91] and memory. It's almost like a puzzle. If you're missing a few pieces, the masterpiece won't look finished. Every piece makes a difference.

---

88 See footnote 87.

89 Suni, E., and Vyas, N. (2022). *Stages of sleep*. Sleep Foundation. https://www.sleepfoundation.org/stages-of-sleep.

90 See footnote 89.

91 Drago, V., Foster, P. S., Heilman, K. M., Aricò, D., Williamson, J., Montagna, P., and Ferri, R. (2011). Cyclic alternating pattern in sleep and its relationship to creativity. *Sleep Medicine, 12*(4), 361-366.

In REM, we notice a lot of brain activity,[92] which means we got a lot going on in this sleep stage. We spend more time in REM sleep toward the latter half of the night as our bodies prepare for its final awakening. This is so that we don't go from a deep stage to just becoming awake out of nowhere. REM happens every 90 to 120 minutes in humans, whereas animals, such as giraffes, spend less than one hour in REM per night.[93] When I saw this giraffe fact, I honestly lost my shit. How do they function off one hour of REM?

Although scientists are still uncovering the function of sleep, specifically REM sleep, we know that we tend to remember our dreams when we are in REM cycles. As we discussed earlier, we are still investigating the meaning of dreams. Our breathing and heart rate tend to increase, and we experience atonia (loss of muscle tone so that we don't act out our dreams) and rapid eye movement while our eyes are closed.[94] Just like the amount of sleep we need changes over time, so does our need for REM sleep.[95] Newborns and babies spend about 50 percent of their time in REM, whereas adults spend about 20 percent in REM.[96] It's crazy how different it is, but sleep changes as we age.

Sleep Stages

Are REM and non-REM friends? Hell yeah, they are besties but don't show up to the party at the same time. They create our human sleep cycle, which lasts approximately ninety minutes and occurs four to

---

92   Peever, J., and Fuller, P. M. (2017). The biology of REM sleep. *Current Biology, 27*(22), R1237-R1248.

93   See footnote 92.

94   National Cancer Institute. (n.d.). *Rapid eye movement sleep.* NCI Dictionaries. https://www.cancer. gov/publications/dictionaries/cancer-terms/def/rapid-eye-movement-sleep.

95   See footnote 92.

96   Daftary, A. S., Jalou, H. E., Shivley, L., Slavens, J. E., and Davis, S. D. (2019). Polysomnography reference values in healthy newborns. *Journal of Clinical Sleep Medicine, 15*(3), 437–443.

five times per night.[97] So if we are getting consolidated sleep (a.k.a. we have few awakenings throughout the night), we can assume that we may be getting into all stages of sleep.[98] In a perfect world (lol, what is perfect?), we're awake, then drift off into N1, N2, N3, then REM sleep. "Normal healthy functioning" adults typically experience about two to three awakenings overnight, which increases as we age.[99] I put this in quotes because I don't know what normal is anymore, as we discussed earlier. Toward the end of the night, we may have these awakenings because our bodies are preparing to wake up completely. However, a few things mess up our sleep cycles.

The first buzzkill for our sleep cycle is alcohol. Yeah, yeah, I know; it may help reduce our sleep latency (a.k.a. the time it takes us to fall asleep). It might feel good to pass out quickly, but it inhibits us from reaching every stage of sleep. It also may delay sleep onset for some people.[100] Alcohol is a central nervous system depressant, which slows our thinking and brain activity, which may cause someone to fall into deeper stages of sleep more quickly. Therefore, it reduces our ability to get enough REM sleep in the beginning of the night, and there might be a rebound effect later.[101] Even though we tend to have more REM sleep in the latter half of the night, it's important to also get what we need at the beginning of the night. We'll chat in-depth about alcohol in a future chapter, but here's a sneak peek.

So, what does our body do with this? Well, it does the best it can with this imbalance, but it may overall affect sleep quality.[102] It's almost like

---

97   See footnote 39.

98   See footnote 82.

99   Johns Hopkins Medicine. (n.d.). *Up in the middle of the night? How to get back to sleep.* https://www.hopkinsmedicine.org/health/wellness-and-prevention/up-in-the-middle-of-the-night-how-to-get-back-to-sleep.

100 Pacheco, D., and Singh, A. (2022). *Alcohol and sleep.* Sleep Foundation. https://www.sleepfoundation.org/nutrition/alcohol-and-sleep.

101 See footnote 100.

102 See footnote 100.

taking medication to put you to sleep. It helps get us there, but our bodies might become confused once it wears off. Alcohol is also a toxin metabolized in the liver, which takes some time. As alcohol leaves the system, our bodies may experience more awakenings.[103] I did a deep dive one time and researched exactly what happens to our bodies when we drink alcohol, and it scared the fuck out of me. It caused me to change a few habits. I never had an issue with alcohol, but I am more curious about my response when someone asks if I want another drink. The answer is usually no. I want my body to work efficiently and have less bullshit to deal with, you know?

"Okay, Kristen, but how much alcohol will really mess up my sleep architecture?" It's hard to say because alcohol is metabolized differently for everyone, based on age, sex, body size, medical conditions, and the amount consumed (and how quickly). These statistics, again, will be binary for men and women and I wish they expanded for nonbinary and trans individuals, but take this as you will. The National Sleep Foundation suggests that one drink for women and two for men impacted sleep quality by 9.3 percent, and more than two drinks for men and more than one drink for women affected sleep quality by 39.2 percent.[104] If you notice a pattern here, the USDA suggests that moderate drinking includes one standard drink for women and two for men per day.[105, 106] This means that any more alcohol than this may have a negative impact on our bodies, and this includes sleep. After writing this I decided to include alcohol in Chapter 5. More on this later because there's too much left unsaid here.

---

103 See footnote 100.

104 See footnote 100.

105 Centers for Disease Control. (2022). *Alcohol and public health.* https://www.cdc.gov/alcohol/index.htm.

106 United States Department of Agriculture. (2020). *Dietary Guidelines for Americans, 2020-2025 and Online Materials.* https://www.dietaryguidelines.gov/resources/2020-2025-dietary-guidelines-online-materials.

Anyway, our body's ability to travel through these sleep stages happens because, well, we're sleepy. We don't usually drift off into sleep if we are simply tired. There are differences here. It's usually a point of contention for people because they may be tired and want to sleep, but that's not what our bodies are asking for. Talking about the differences is helpful so that you don't expect something of your body that you're not capable of at the time.

Tiredness vs. Sleepiness

I tell my clients that **sleep is for restoration, not relaxation**. Read that again. Sleep isn't technically super useful if we're simply tired; it's usually indicated for when we are sleepy. Yes, there are differences here. I mean, sure, sleep off your problems; sometimes we want to just check out. But if we do this every time we are tired, we might not be addressing the issue at hand. I know these might seem like subtle differences, but this is important as you evaluate your sleep health and habits because you might be working hard to sleep and still feel exhausted (work smarter, not harder).

If you are using sleep for relaxation or avoidance and waking up exhausted and anxious, it's probably because sleep wasn't what your body needed. So, knowing these subtle differences and some of the science behind sleep is useful to know what your body needs. This knowledge reduces the confusion so you can focus more energy on dealing with other things, such as a big work project or taking care of your kids.

Tiredness means that our bodies are physically shot. Maybe your muscles hurt or your brain is exhausted. You worked all day and can't think straight, and you need to simply exist and not have any more input. You might lie on the couch and be unable to fall asleep, but your body is like, "Nope, it's a no from me. We don't want to sleep right now." What the hell are we supposed to do with that? Doesn't sleep fix everything? Nope.

There's also this concept of your soul being tired. It's when you feel burnt out with life or don't have a sense of meaning or purpose. You feel disconnected to the people closest to you. You might be tired of doing the same thing every day. Your body is sluggish like there's no pep in your step. Sleep doesn't fix when your soul is tired, when you're burnt out at work, if your partner's infidelity is eating away at you, or if your family doesn't accept your sexuality, even after decades of convincing. The concept of sleepiness is different.

When we are very sleepy, it means our body's sleep drive is high. Sleep drive is technically the body's biological need for sleep.[107] Every hour you're awake, your body's sleep drive increases (pretty cool, right?). Your sleep drive is low when you wake up in the morning because you slept all night. This means that your body's biological need for sleep is low, and it's less likely that you'll need sleep immediately upon waking. Your sleep drive and circadian rhythm usually go together here because your body also needs signals from your circadian rhythm, a.k.a. your suprachiasmatic nucleus (SCN), which also promotes wakefulness and sleepiness. In the CBT-I protocol, we use the hunger drive analogy to compare to sleep drive. If you just ate a piece of cake, your hunger drive decreases.[108] Therefore, it's less likely that you're hungry. It's the same with our body's sleep drive.

107 De Valck, E, and Cluydts, R. (2003). Sleepiness as a state-trait phenomenon, comprising both a sleep drive and a wake drive. *Medical Hypotheses, 60*(4), 509–512.

108 Espie, C.A. (2022). Standard CBT-I protocol for the treatment of insomnia disorder. In *Cognitive-behavioural therapy for insomnia (CBT-I) across the life span* (eds C. Baglioni, C.A. Espi, D. Riemann, , and). https://doi.org/10.1002/9781119891192.ch2

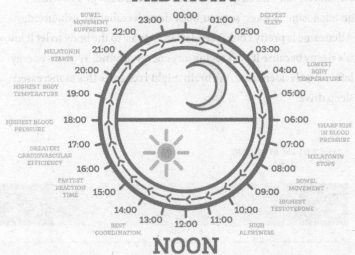

So, I know you're wondering, "What the hell *is* sleep drive? Is it like an organ? A part of the brain?" Not necessarily. Here's a super simplified version of the inner workings of sleep drive. I say this because, again, there are plenty of resources that talk about this in a complex way, and this book is designed to make these concepts digestible and practical so that you can remember them easily when working on your sleep health.

In a nutshell: Adenosine is a nucleotide in most of our cells that lets our bodies know we're sleepy. There is a slow buildup of adenosine and a reduction of energy as our day progresses.[109] Adenosine is a

---

[109] Huang, Z., Urade, Y., and Hayaishi, O. (2011). The role of adenosine in the regulation of sleep. *Current Topics in Medicinal Chemistry, 11*(8), 1047–1057.

consequence of burning energy, so the more our energy is depleted, the more exhausted we feel. Napping is an energy-restoring activity, so it reduces the effects of adenosine so our bodies don't feel tired anymore. And that large iced coffee you're drinking? Yeah, that's an adenosine blocker, so your body doesn't realize it's exhausted. Adenosine is pretty cool; it sends flare signals to the body to let it know it's sleepy because it isn't seeing any energy around. With no energy left and only adenosine, the brain might recognize this as increased sleep drive.

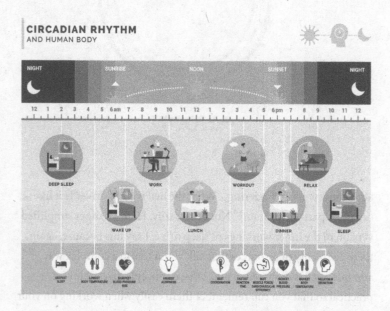

CIRCADIAN RHYTHM
AND HUMAN BODY

Of course, this is an example of someone's circadian rhythm if they woke up at the same time each day. Our body knows what to expect, and everyone's needs are different. My peak coordination time may differ from yours because we wake up at different times and have different biological needs.

Sleepiness means our bodies need, well, sleep. Tiredness means we need to relax, meditate, and reorganize our thoughts. Being awake and existing without input for the sake of meditating and sleep have different functions for our body. In my opinion, if we're tired and attempt to sleep, we might be trying to avoid the things causing the tiredness in the first place. Yeah, you might simply be tired from working all day. But how are you *really* doing? Tiredness, especially that deep sense of exhaustion unrelated to our sleep health, is a silent buzzkill for the quality of our life. We might feel beaten down at work, not good enough in our relationship, or stressed about equal rights or reproductive health policies. It's a heavy burden to carry. You might also be tired of doing this damn thing every day. Nothing feels exciting. Sleep won't fix that, and introspection and therapy might help you come to other conclusions about how to live a more meaningful and fulfilling life with the cards you're dealt.

Internal and External Cues for Sleepiness

"But what if I still can't tell the difference?" That's okay; you're here to learn, not to know everything. We can tell the difference between sleepiness and tiredness in a few ways. The most notable one for me is becoming more aware of our internal bodily cues for sleepiness, including drowsiness, yawning, or nodding off while watching television. If you can't even stay awake, that lets you know that your body needs sleep. If you are exhausted but can probably get behind the wheel of a car, you're likely tired. External cues also let our bodies know that we're tired, which might be easier to pick up on. This includes the time of day, bedtime routine, or exposure to light.

Well, now that we're on the subject, our sleep drive and circadian rhythm work together to help us drift off to sleep. Think about being exhausted and sleep (sleep drive) and it's dark out and your body feels ready for sleep (circadian rhythm). Again, an oversimplified version of this, but our circadian rhythm helps to regulate our sleep-wake cycle, a.k.a. when we fall asleep and when we wake up. So, if we wake up at the same time every day and expose ourselves to light immediately upon waking, our body knows it's show time. We're ready to go. It's the same when light goes away. If you notice, during Daylight Saving Time, it gets darker earlier, and most people report feeling a bit sleepier once the sun goes down. Our bodies use this as an external cue to regulate our cycle.

Okay, so what *is* a circadian rhythm? Well, circadian rhythms help our bodies regulate certain processes within a twenty-four-hour cycle. It's like a biological manager of our mental, behavioral, and physical processes.[110] The manager ensures that certain activities take place so we're the most effective and efficient humans. It tries to make things happen around the same time every day for consistency, such as melatonin secretion. If we don't have consistency, this manager has to work harder against our sleep expectations. If we wake up at nine o'clock one day and eleven o'clock the next day, our manager initiates certain processes and functions based on the time that we wake up, so we might not have those internal cues of sleepiness until later than expected. However, if we wake up at nine o'clock every day, we can expect our bodies to become tired around the same time, so we aren't sitting up awake and frustrated in bed.

These circadian rhythms are connected to a biological clock. Our sleep-wake cycle is one circadian rhythm, located in the suprachiasmatic nucleus (SCN) within the hypothalamus.[111] Our SCN is extremely sensitive to the external cue of light and thrives off

---

110 Sollars, P. J., and Pickard, G. E. (2015). The neurobiology of circadian rhythms. *Psychiatric Clinics*, *38*(4), 645–665.

111 National Institute of General Medical Sciences. (2022). *Circadian rhythms*. https://www.nigms.nih. gov/education/fact-sheets/Pages/circadian-rhythms.aspx.

a consistent wake time. Like, super sensitive. Almost like if you have a severe peanut allergy and cannot even be in the same room as peanuts. So, when it's bright outside, our SCN sends signals to our body to stay alert and awake.[112] Once the sun leaves, our body produces melatonin, which helps the body start the orchestrated events that promote sleepiness. Melatonin is secreted throughout the night, letting the body know we can stay asleep.

As you can see, sleepiness has a certain function and effect on our bodies compared to tiredness. Our bodies don't need sleep when we are tired; they might simply need to relax and engage the parasympathetic nervous system (our relaxation response).[113] Achieving somewhat of a meditative state or engaging in mindfulness practices helps to promote a relaxation response.[114] If you're sleepy, you sleep. If you're tired, you rest your brain and body. We also know that these relaxation strategies may help promote sleepiness for those who are anxious or stressed.[115] Not to be a buzzkill, but we have to talk about poor sleep. It sucks, we've all experienced it, and I want to dive right in because we gotta rip the Band-Aid off here.

Poor Sleep

So, you've seen the terms "poor sleep," "sleep deprivation," "sleep deficiency," and "insomnia," among other sleep-related issues. What are the differences? There are plenty of nuances here.

112 Healthy Sleep. (2017). *Under the brain's control*. Division of Sleep Medicine at Harvard Medical School. https://healthysleep.med.harvard.edu/healthy/science/how/neurophysiology.

113 Wikipedia. (2020). *The relaxation response*. http://sagecraft-lifecoach.org/wp-content/uploads/2020/08/0000.-The_Relaxation_Response.pdf.

114 Tang, Y. Y., Ma, Y., Fan, Y., Feng, H., Wang, J., Feng, S., Lu, Q., Hu, B., Lin, Y., Li, J., Zhang, Y., Wang, Y., Zhou, L., and Fan, M. (2009). Central and autonomic nervous system interaction is altered by short-term meditation. *Proceedings of the National Academy of Sciences, 106*(22), 8865-8870.

115 Nagendra, R. P., Maruthai, N., and Kutty, B. M. (2012). Meditation and its regulatory role on sleep. *Frontiers in Neurology, 3*, 54.

Just for background, there are so many sleep disorders. There are
over seventy of them (audible gasp!). Most psychologists use the
Diagnostic and Statistical Manual of Mental Disorders (DSM-5).
The DSM has different categories of sleep-wake disorders, including
insomnia, hypersomnolence, narcolepsy, breathing-related sleep
disorders, circadian rhythm sleep-wake disorders, non-rapid eye
movement (NREM) sleep arousal disorders, nightmare disorder, rapid
eye movement (REM) sleep behavior disorder, restless leg syndrome,
and substance/medication-induced sleep disorder.[116] Most of these
disorders involve poor sleep or issues with regulating sleep, so let's
start with the basics.

A poor night of sleep might be defined as difficulty falling or staying
asleep, which results in fragmented sleep cycles. We might not get
into those deep stages of sleep or get enough REM sleep, which helps
our bodies with certain functions. Poor quality sleep breaches the
threshold of chronic insomnia when we experience difficulty falling
or staying asleep, dissatisfaction with the quality of our sleep, and
waking up before our intended alarm without an ability to fall back to
sleep at least three times per week for about three months. So in short,
if you experience a shitty night of sleep three times per week for three
months, it might be time to look deeply into your sleep health. It also
may be situational, and once the stressor passes, your sleep health
might return to baseline. Either way, it's not a bad idea to become
curious about your sleep health.

Many people view sleep deprivation as an overall loss of hours of
sleep over days or weeks. Some use an hourly cutoff to classify it
as less than six or seven hours of sleep per night. Others view sleep
deprivation as sleeping the recommended amount of sleep, but having

---

116 American Psychiatric Association. *Diagnostic and statistical manual of mental disorders*, 5th ed.
     Arlington: American Psychiatric Association, 2013.

many awakenings that disrupt sleep architecture. Sleep deprivation is a blanket term that many laypeople use to describe sleep as "I'm straight-up not having a great time, and I'm exhausted all the time." I know you know what this feels like because I can easily recall what this feels like for me. Walking from my bedroom to the kitchen feels exhausting because I can't function, and my body is yelling at me to stay in bed.

Sleep Deprivation or Insomnia?

Most of us view sleep deprivation as a chronic issue. And this is partially correct. Acute sleep deprivation accounts for a significant reduction in sleep time for a few days. On the other hand, chronic sleep deprivation lasts for three months or longer.[117] We are looking at hours here (a.k.a. sleep time). However, The American Academy of Sleep Medicine (AASM) suggests using sleep deficiency or insufficiency are more helpful terms than sleep deprivation because it accounts for the time lost while sleeping (a.k.a. the hours of sleep lost).[118] I like when concepts are refined this way because it helps us know what we're looking at and how we can overcome it.

How the hell is sleep deprivation different from insomnia? Nuanced once again, but important differences because they both may be treated differently. Both involve not getting enough quality sleep. An easy way to remember insomnia is that those with insomnia don't sleep well even when they have opportunities to sleep. Those with sleep deprivation *don't* have an opportunity to sleep because of life obligations or things that get in the way. Sleep deprivation is usually a result of life obligations that get in the way of prioritizing sleep,

---

117 See footnote 66.

118 National Heart, Lung, and Blood Institute. (2022). *What are sleep deprivation and deficiency?* U.S. Department of Health and Human Services. https://www.nhlbi.nih.gov/health/sleep-deprivation.

whereas insomnia involves difficulty falling or staying asleep, waking up before your intended alarm, and overall dissatisfaction with sleep despite having an opportunity to sleep.[119] Insomnia may involve issues with your sleep drive, heightened arousal, or a circadian rhythm that is misaligned with our preferred bed/wake times.

Picture this: Dominique has a bed window of eight hours. This means that she's dedicated eight of her hours to sleep. She struggles to fall asleep, and when she does, she may have frequent awakenings. These awakenings last pretty long because she's thinking about all of the embarrassing moments in her life. Her total sleep time may be six hours, but her bed window is eight hours. She has the time allocated for eight hours regardless. Jai has a bed window of five hours. They may or may not experience difficulty falling or staying asleep, but they have less opportunity to gain sleep hours. They work until eight in the evening and wake up at five o'clock, but they usually binge Netflix until midnight. So who has insomnia and who has sleep deprivation?

Yep, Dominique may have insomnia and Jai may experience sleep deprivation. It also depends on the person. Some people operate a little better with less than eight hours; others need more than eight hours of rest to feel ready for the day. If you have siblings, think about your sleep needs; they might vary. I know I operate well with a little less than seven hours, whereas my brother needs more sleep than me to function effectively.

Whether we technically have insomnia, sleep deficiency/insufficiency, or poor sleep, it may occur for various reasons. It can be due to sleep apnea, life obligations, chronic stress, lifestyle choices, medical issues, or other psychological issues, such as anxiety or depression.[120] They

---

119 Suni, E., and Rehman, A. (2022). *Insomnia*. Sleep Foundation. https://www.sleepfoundation.org/insomnia.

120 See footnote 56.

both include potentially feeling sleepy during the day. People may also experience what we call microsleeps, which are short episodes (one to fifteen seconds) when we doze off[121] because we are exhausted. This can be caused by sleep deprivation, insomnia, or narcolepsy. However, not everyone who experiences microsleeps has narcolepsy, a rare neurological condition where someone experiences sleep attacks because of the brain's inability to regulate sleep/wake cycles.[122, 123] These people may experience microsleeps regardless of how long they've slept the day before. Regardless of the cause, the consequences of not getting enough quality sleep can be detrimental if we don't take action.

Consequences of Poor Sleep

We've chatted about the function of sleep, why it's important, and how far we've come in the sleep medicine world. We know what poor sleep is, but what happens as a result of poor sleep? Well, where do you want me to begin? The TLDR: it has the potential to wreck your well-being and health over time if you don't pay attention to it and make even slight changes to enhance the quality of your sleep.

I always thought I could "catch up" on sleep. If I had a rough week, I'd just sleep more on the weekends. I should be good after that, right? Ah, not so much. I was so angry when I read this statistic online. Yes, you might feel better after sleeping on the weekends, but it doesn't effectively heal the time we lost.

---

121 Poudel, G. R., Innes, C. R. H., Bones, P. J., Watts, R., and Jones, R. D. (2012). Losing the struggle to stay awake: Divergent thalamic and cortical activity during microsleeps. *Human Brain Mapping*, *35*, 257-269.

122 Lights, V., and Boskey, E. (2022). *Narcolepsy*. Healthline. https://www.healthline.com/health/narcolepsy.

123 National Institute of Neurological Disorders and Stroke. (2022). *Fact sheets*. U.S. Department of Health and Human Services. https://www.ninds.nih.gov/health-information/patient-caregiver-education/fact-sheets.

The research shows that if we have accumulated sleep debt, we can't effectively catch up on the sleep we lost in the days prior.[124] For example, one study suggested trying to catch up on sleep isn't a helpful strategy because it doesn't reverse weight gain from lost sleep or the metabolic dysregulation caused by lack of sleep throughout the week.[125] Sleep debt is basically like a debt you can't pay back with sleeping more. You have to exist with the consequences of your actions or actions outside your control.

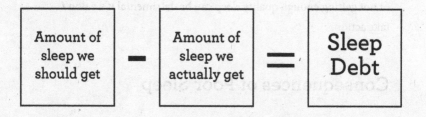

RIP to all of those hours lost, or should we say RIS? Rest in Sleep? Anyway… What happens to our bodies when we have insomnia, poor sleep, or sleep deficiency or insufficiency? Well, it depends on how long these have been going on. The consequences for someone with acute insomnia (insomnia that happens for a few weeks) might look different than someone with chronic insomnia (insomnia for more than three months). It also may be different for someone with untreated sleep apnea (episodes of non-breathing that result in a lack of oxygen to the brain). I will generalize here because there are so many sleep disorders and endless ways that sleep can become dysregulated.

124 Newsom, R., and Rehman, A. (2022). *Sleep debt and catching up on sleep*. Sleep Foundation. https://www.sleepfoundation.org/how-sleep-works/sleep-debt-and-catch-up-sleep.

125 Depner, C. M., Melanson, E. L., Eckel, R. H., Snell-Bergeon, J. K., Perreault, L., Bergman, B. C., Higgins, J. A., Guerin, M. K., Stothard, E. R., Morton, S. J., and Wright Jr., K. P. (2019). *Ad libitum* weekend recovery sleep fails to prevent metabolic dysregulation during a repeating pattern of insufficient sleep and weekend recovery sleep. *Current Biology, 29*(6), 957–967.

We know that sleep helps with cognition, memory consolidation, growth and development, performance, involuntary metabolic processes, such as temperature and cellular regulation, muscle, cell, and tissue repair, and more. Sleep deprivation may cause weight gain, memory issues, concentration and attention difficulties, irritability or mood issues, low sex drive, or weakened immune system. It also may cause increased absenteeism, accidents, poor performance, and increased use of medications or doctor's visits. We may be at higher risk for medical issues, such as high blood pressure or diabetes.[126] All this happens because we *don't* prioritize sleep? Think about all the shit that happens to us even if we are sleeping well.

We may already be at risk for health conditions based on our genetics and sleep issues may make this worse. That's why sleep is so important. A lot is working against you just by being a human alive on this earth. Being alive is a lot of work, for real. Finding the controllable factors related to sleep is where our power is. Saying things like, "Oh yeah, I just suck at sleep" or "This is just the way I am," might not get you closer to a good night's sleep; it may be causing more harm because we don't take accountability for the controllables that impact our sleep. I think it's helpful to acknowledge the starting point by saying these things, but taking action is important.

The Sleep Debt Cycle

Think about what happens to you when you don't get enough sleep or your sleep is fragmented. Let's look at two scenarios. You wake up and say, "Wow, did I get hit by a train? Did I even sleep? Am I going to make it through today? I'm exhausted." You call off from work and try

126 Watson, S., and Cherney, K. (2021). *The effects of sleep deprivation on your body.* Healthline. https://www.healthline.com/health/sleep-deprivation/effects-on-body.

to sleep in. Calling off is difficult because you already feel uneasy about asking people to use your pronouns and name different from your driver's license. You might drink more coffee than usual or go to the doctor because you feel sick or ill. Maybe you take ibuprofen for that pounding headache or try to do something productive around your house but you're ineffective. You can't justify paying a babysitter when you're home, so your kids want to do fun things. You can barely figure out how to muster up the energy to feed them a good meal, so you pull out whatever is in the freezer. Then, the shame cycle begins. "Why can't I just get it together? Why am I like this?" Then, you turn on the news. Not only is your life spiraling, but millions of people are dealing with horrible things that you wish you could change. Maybe you're an advocate for these things. You might be ineffective today because of your sleep and can't help yourself or those around you.

If you don't have the privilege of calling off of work, your day might look like this: You look at your alarm clock or watch, audibly gasp, curse a little, try to sleep in as long as you can, then begrudgingly get out of bed. You barely throw yourself together and make it to work a little later than usual. You arrive at work, exhausted and irritable, wanting to cry from feeling so out of it. Maybe your coworkers call you out on your vibe, which is another reminder that you couldn't sleep. You're already irritable so any little thing at work causes intense frustration (we've all been there). Then, the obligatory and painful thought patterns begin. *When I get home, I have to clean the house and pick up the kids, and not only that, but they might want to do something. What am I supposed to do if I'm exhausted? I also have to drive home that weird way, which makes me feel unsafe, ah, everything sucks.* You start to imagine what the day will look like after work, and it becomes overwhelming.

In either situation, you might try to lie down for a nap at your first opportunity. Then, you're up all night because your sleep drive isn't high by the time you lie down at midnight, and now your circadian rhythm is fucked. Then, it starts all over again. I'm sure you can see that one night of poor sleep can wreck your next day, but think about this as your norm. This might be your norm. You might read this like, "Shit, that's me." Think about how unintentional everything is, from waking up in a panic to barely getting dressed to maybe calling off work or trying to do your job. Either way, you're ineffective in multiple areas of life and you're not an active participant in your life.

These scenarios are the tip of the iceberg for some people. We aren't accounting for day-to-day stress, or chronic systemic stress that comes from discrimination, inequality, or racial oppression. The stress that you can't fix. The stress that you can't do much about. We aren't here to fix the system because we can only do so much. We can acknowledge that the system causes uncontrollable stressful experiences. We can validate our experiences and notice that these situations impact our stress. Then, we focus on the small things we can do to help ourselves sleep better or prioritize sleep differently.

That might mean prioritizing sleep health, reducing caffeine, or seeing a therapist for stress management strategies. And let's not underestimate the power of leveling with our friends or partner to vent about our stress and gain support during tough times. If you aren't the talker, you might ask friends to spend more time with you, hit up a comedy club, go for an intense nature walk, or sit and cry to help the feelings surface. A good cry never hurt anybody!

Real Talk: Sleep Deprivation Edition

What happens every hour without sleep? Well, a lot. Every person may experience this differently, but let's talk about the general issues when it comes to losing much-needed sleep on a daily basis. Have you ever stayed up because of a road trip or because you've had a lot of work to do? Maybe you're traveling and you've been awake on an international flight for over twenty-four hours. Maybe you're experiencing stress and it's difficult to find the time to sleep. Or maybe you have shift work and chose a shift directly after your traditional shift, causing you to be awake for a day or two.

A lot happens when we sleep, and there are a lot of consequences when we don't sleep. If you're the type to stay up for a few days at a time or you're wondering what happens to your brain and body when you're sleep-deprived, stay tuned.

Before we get into the hour-by-hour timeline, I'll give you an idea of what happens to our bodies when sleep-deprived. We're less likely to be efficient when fighting off infections, and our immune system functioning may take a hit.[127] We likely need to prioritize our sleep when we do become ill because our bodies desperately want to fight off the infections we have. Have you ever had the flu and noticed you're sluggish and just want to sleep? Sleep helps restore our immune system functioning, and sleep deprivation might make this difficult.

Our Immune System Tanks

I like to see the immune system as your body's army. It's on standby for any attackers that infiltrate your body, and your immune system is designed to keep your body alive and free of foreign attackers. If your army is too tired to fight, what happens to you? Nobody else is doing this job; it's not like you have a backup immune system that can step in and be as active or helpful as your primary immune system. You can't

---

127 Asif, N., Iqbal, R., and Nazir, C. F. (2017). Human immune system during sleep. *American Journal of Clinical and Experimental Immunology, 6*(6), 92-96.

call your friend and be like, "Hey, man, can I borrow your immune system for a bit? I'm fucking exhausted." Then your friend has no immune system…you see where this is going.

Heart Struggles

Our cardiovascular system also suffers when we experience sleep deprivation. Sleep deprivation increases our risk for hypertension, cardiovascular arrhythmias, and coronary artery disease,[128, 129] a.k.a. the things that we don't want to happen to our heart. The heart works twenty-four seven and it is basically our lifeline. If our hearts aren't functioning properly, that's likely to affect everything, including brain function. Our brains rely on receiving oxygenated blood to function. You see where I'm going with this. Not to mention, we only have one heart. It's not like the liver, where it has the potential to regenerate. We have one shot at this, and we should treat our hearts kindly because it's the muscle that doesn't stop. It never has the opportunity for a break. And if it does take a break, well, see ya.

Cancer Ain't Fun

Sleep deprivation, or shortened sleep, also increases our risk of developing certain types of cancer, including breast and prostate

---

128 Tobaldini, E., Costantino, G., Solbiati, M., Cogliati, C., Kara, T., Nobili, L., and Montano, N. (2017). Sleep, sleep deprivation, autonomic nervous system and cardiovascular diseases. *Neuroscience & Biobehavioral Reviews, 74*(B), 321-329.

129 Mullington, J. M., Haack, M., Toth, M., Serrador, J. M., and Meier-Ewert, H. K. (2009). Cardiovascular, inflammatory, and metabolic consequences of sleep deprivation. *Progress in Cardiovascular Diseases, 51*(4), 294-302.

cancer[130] and stomach and esophageal cancers.[131] I think about how our stomach and digestive systems are so incredibly important. Our body's way of digesting food is so important for our health. Not to mention how sleep affects cancer relating to our primary sex characteristics (e.g., breasts in cisgender women and penises in cisgender men). This may affect our livelihood and sense of belonging as it relates to our sexual and gender identities. As you can see, it's easy to say, "lack of sleep increases our risk of cancer," but it's important to understand what this means and what can be at stake. Our sex characteristics guide how we experience the world and view our sexual and gender identities. They're pretty important.

Hot Sex or No?

Let's talk more about sex and how sleep deprivation affects our sex lives. Sleep deprivation can affect our libido, a fancy word for sexual desire. It's how excited we are about engaging in intimacy. Attraction and desire are two separate concepts, and I like to focus on desire when I think of libido because sexual experiences can also be solo activities. We've seen that those who experience sleep deprivation also have a noticeable decrease in sex hormones, such as testosterone, for cisgender men.[132] I know we sometimes relate testosterone only to reproduction, but it's also important for bone density, muscle mass, and strength.[133]

130 Mogavero, M. P., DelRosso, L. M., Fanfulla, F., Bruni, O., and Ferri, R. (2021). Sleep disorders and cancer: State of the art and future perspectives. *Sleep Medicine Reviews, 56,* 101409.

131 Brzecka, A., Sarul, K., Dyła, T., Avila-Rodriguez, M., Cabezas-Perez, R., Chubarev, V. N., Minyaeva, N. N., Klochkov, S. G., Neganova, M. E., Mikhaleva, L. M., Somasundaram, S. G., Kirkland, C. E., Tarasov, V. V., and Aliev, G. (2020). The association of sleep disorders, obesity and sleep-related hypoxia with cancer. *Current Genomics, 21*(6), 444–453.

132 Leproult, R., and Van Cauter, E. (2011). Effect of 1 week of sleep restriction on testosterone levels in young healthy men. *JAMA, 305*(21), 2173–2174.

133 Bremner, W. J. (2010). Testosterone deficiency and replacement in older men. *The New England Journal of Medicine, 363*(2), 189-191.

Sleep Affects Our Body Weight

Sleep deprivation also affects our weight. I'm not going to suggest sleeping better for weight loss. In my mind, weight loss is never the goal. Body shape and weight concerns are usually something we notice because we are taught unrealistic beauty standards and expectations by a system that benefits from our insecurities. Damn, too deep? Weight gain may simply tell us something isn't right with our bodies. I *sometimes* like to use it as a measurement to help us figure out if our bodies are operating up to par. If you're used to fluctuating three to five pounds per day, but you're noticing way more or less, it might be a sign to think about your sleep health.

Researchers suggest there's a link between short sleep and weight gain, suggesting that those who sleep less than five hours per night are more likely to experience this weight gain.[134] Think about the effect of short sleep duration over the course of years. Maybe your goal is to have a healthier lifestyle and incorporate movement into your daily routine. Well, this is helpful, but if you're using the scale to dictate your progress, it's likely that sleep (or lack thereof) also influences this outcome. Sometimes weight gain can indicate poor health conditions, but it doesn't always equate to being unhealthy. Important difference here. When I think of weight gain in the sleep realm, I use it as a data point to suggest our sleep may be suffering in some way. The key is getting better quality sleep rather than trying to lose weight. If we try to lose weight, we might overlook the origin of this issue, and our weight loss journey may not fix the entire problem. So, if you're a provider reading this, let's focus on the reasons for weight gain other than poor eating habits because there's more to it than that.

---

134 Kobayashi, D., Takahashi, O., Deshpande, G. A., Shimbo, T., and Fukui, T. (2012). Association between weight gain, obesity, and sleep duration: A large-scale 3-year cohort study. *Sleep and Breathing, 16*, 829–833.

Is Your Skin Glowing or Lifeless?

Ah, we can't talk about the effects of sleep deprivation without acknowledging its effect on our skin. If there's anything that can convince you to get more sleep, maybe it's your looks. An interesting study conducted in 2020 examined the effects of sleep deprivation for thirty Korean women in their forties.[135] Researchers measured factors from hydration to texture to gloss, and they also included frown lines, crow's feet, and skin color. The women slept eight hours per night for the first week and then four hours per night for the second week. I'd probably cry if I was a part of this study, but the participants consented to this, and it wasn't a chronic sleep deprivation experiment over the course of years, so they should be okay.

Ready for the skin results? This had me flabbergasted, to say the least. Researchers found that sleep-deprived women were more likely to experience skin dehydration after *one* day of sleep deprivation. One. ✋ Day. ✋ They also explained that gloss, elasticity, and wrinkles intensified after one day of sleep deprivation. They didn't notice much with skin texture after one day, but elasticity was the most notable characteristic that changed over time.[136] Isn't this wild? Skin is technically our biggest organ, and it makes sense that it would be affected in some way.

We know that maintaining our skin barrier might be an uphill battle. We are up against sun exposure, pollutants, harmful makeup ingredients, and more. Just like we use sunscreen or pure makeup ingredients, we can preventatively help our skin health by prioritizing sleep. In fact, some dermatologists suggest that our skin also operates

---

135 Jang, S. I., Lee, M., Han, J., Kim, J., Kim, A. R., An, J. S., Park, J. O., Kim, B. J., and Kim, E. (2020). A study of skin characteristics with long-term sleep restriction in Korean women in their 40s. *Skin Research and Technology, 26*(2), 193–199.

136 See footnote 134.

on a circadian rhythm similar to our sleep cycle.[137] They call it a cutaneous circadian system (cutaneous is the biological term for skin). Our skin is our body's biggest organ and repairs itself at night.[138]

I'm sure dermatologists can suggest certain products to assist our skin's overnight repair process. And prioritizing your sleep is free. It might be challenging to prioritize, but it's not as much of a financial burden as upping our skincare regimen. Not all of us have the money to buy the latest products that cost as much as filling our gas tank.

Sleep Deprivation: Hour by Hour

Okay, now for the grand finale for sleep deprivation. What happens hour by hour? During the first twenty-four hours of no sleep, you might notice drowsiness, fatigue, lack of coordination and energy, mood issues such as irritability and stress, and you might be prone to more accidents or making mistakes. You might also crave certain foods and experience dark circles under your eyes (who wants that?). Think about how you overcome these experiences—by compensating for them. You might use more makeup, drink more energy drinks, and generally eat more. And this isn't free. You pay for food, drinks, and makeup with the money you make at the job that makes you exhausted. It's a vicious cycle, right?

Then, thirty-six hours with no sleep means these symptoms feel a lot worse. Spoiler alert: it's only downhill from here. Buckle up, baby—everything gets worse until this chapter ends, so keep reading if you want to know the stone-cold truth. (I laughed as I wrote this.)

---

137 Matsui, M. S., Pelle, E., Dong, K., and Pernodet, N. (2016). Biological rhythms in the skin. *International Journal of Molecular Sciences, 17*(6), 801.

138 See footnote 136.

Anyway, you might be even more groggy than yesterday and experience short bursts of sleep (a.k.a. microsleeps). Your body is more likely to be inflamed and your immune system is on its way to check out. You might have issues having conversations or communicating with your coworkers or family members. It's likely that you will forget things or have trouble remembering certain parts of conversations. You might struggle to get your words out (e.g., expressive language issues) or misunderstand what people say (e.g., receptive language). It'll be tough to make decisions, plan things, or react to certain situations, which leads me to believe that our prefrontal cortex is stressed. Our prefrontal cortex—the CEO of our brain, remember?— likes to make decisions and plan stuff. Well, after thirty-six hours of no sleep, our CEO has suffered and needs a break.

What about two days of no sleep, a.k.a. forty-eight hours? Well, shit, it's going to get a little slippery here. This is known as extreme sleep deprivation; it's really difficult to stay awake. If you're ever behind the wheel of a car during this time, I strongly suggest you have someone else drive or get into a rideshare situation. You may experience hallucinations (seeing things that aren't there) or depersonalization, which feels like your body isn't your body. You might feel like you're an outside observer of your body.

Three days of no sleep, a.k.a. seventy-two hours: How the hell are you still awake? I'm sure you're asking yourself that question. Again, all the symptoms highlighted above become more intense. Some people start noticing frightening hallucinations and question what's real and what isn't. Sometimes you might notice delusions, too, which are fixed beliefs that aren't rooted in reality. There are many categories of delusions, but an extreme example might be that your boss is trying to poison you through the food that's offered at your job (persecutory delusions). Or you might believe you will be the next president of the United States, even though you're a sales representative for a company and have never thought about running for office (delusions of grandeur). Of course, these may be real experiences, but they're questionable with no history of these beliefs of this with adequate sleep and there's no evidence to suggest this is happening. It can make reality confusing. You can imagine how confusing this is for you and everyone around you. It's almost hard to trust yourself and your mind at this point.

After ninety-six hours, this reality testing gets worse. Reality testing is a concept therapists sometimes use to help people regain control of their reality during situations like this. It's hard to determine what's real and what's fake, and your body is screaming for sleep. You might experience sleep deprivation psychosis, hallucinations or delusions resulting from lack of sleep. This goes away once you're able to get sleep. As you can see, the symptoms worsen as your body continues to experience no sleep. And, as always, not everyone has these exact symptoms, but they are pretty common for those who experience sleep loss to this degree.

How scary is this? Our bodies react pretty seriously to lack of sleep, hour by hour and day by day. But my problem with this: sleep deprivation has become so normalized in society that we sometimes overlook how detrimental it really is. If you're a night-shift worker, have multiple jobs, are in school, experience a ton of pain, and can't handle your chronic stress, it's likely that you've been a survivor of sleep deprivation. If there are controllables, we handle those; if not, we change our expectations for our bodies. But if we're normalizing this, it's less likely that we will take action. So, the next time you want to pull an all-nighter, ask yourself, "Is there another option for me here?" If not, you gotta do what you gotta do!

So, Why Care?

Because you only get one shot at this and a lot is working against you.

If you're in your twenties, you have some time. If you're in your fifties, you have some time. If you're in your seventies, you have some time. Remember, you can't catch up on sleep, so don't worry about the days, months, or years you've already lost. We can't go back but we can figure out where to go from here. And "here" might be right now, as you're reading this book and deciding to make changes. Toward the end of this book, I will give you the nuts and bolts of what to focus on, which might make it a little easier to implement. But as you continue reading, think about how you might make small changes based on what you've read. They don't have to be enormous changes; even being curious about your sleep is one step.

If the research above isn't enough evidence for you, let's chat about the human experience in raw form. Depending on what you believe, we only get one shot at this whole living thing. You can't go back and redo things. You can't catch up on sleep. You can't go back and be born as someone with a different life. You can't undo the trauma that caused your sleep issues. You can't change much about the past; you can only choose (with limitations, of course) where you go from here. And, even if you make active choices, many things are outside of your control, as we discussed. You might as well figure out what you can have control over, which might be aspects of your sleep.

"Well, this is fucking depressing." Tell me about it. And it shows us that focusing on the small things we can control is so important. If we chalk all of this up to, "It's out of my control," we reduce our ability to enhance our sleep even a little. We've seen that even a small increase in sleep efficiency is helpful for people. Even an increase of one hour of sleep per night helps so much. Do you feel different if you get five hours of sleep versus six? I know I can notice some differences. On five hours of sleep, I'm like, "Oh, screw this," and on six hours, I'm like, "Screw this a little bit." That matters. Let's start to be intentional because life can be a wild ride.

I've followed Buddhism for about eighteen years and spend a good chunk of my time meditating and thinking about certain concepts, like karma and reincarnation. I don't consider myself an expert, nor do I even identify as a Buddhist, because it takes away from those who dedicate their entire lives to this practice. There are a few things from my travels within Buddhism that may relate to sleep, so we can use these as examples of how to apply your spirituality or religion to sleep concepts. For simplicity, the push is to be a good person because that may determine the fundamentals of your next life. You might think, *Oh yeah, my bad karma in this life is poor sleep because maybe I was a dick in a previous life.* Well, that's what I thought about myself initially. I wonder who I was in a previous life, and if I got attacked by needles because I have a needle phobia now.

Anyway, if we think about reincarnation, our soul technically has an opportunity for another chance at life, depending on our specific circumstances. If I get another shot, why care about sleep now? Well, you might continue to have these issues regardless of where you go. Another general concept of Buddhism is that suffering is inevitable. If I had to choose, I'd rather come to terms with the uncontrollable suffering, even if I disagree. Acceptance means coming to terms with it and ending the war in your mind. Acceptance is different than agreeing with your current situation. It's knowing your starting point, even if you desperately want to change it or stop it from happening. Then, you can reduce suffering for the things within your control, like how you view sleep and prioritize it.

You might be spiritual or religious, and I'd suggest leaning into these experiences as they relate to sleep. If you're not either of these things, no worries; totally not mandatory to get good sleep health.

It's also easier for me to think about the controllables in my life because of obvious reasons: I'm a psychologist, so I've had my fair share of therapy and evaluating my life, so I'm used to evaluating these things, and I'm here to help you do the same. This is a privilege within itself that I'm hoping to share more knowledge on—and sometimes your controllables might look different than mine. And your controllables might also look different from those of your partner, kids, friends, or family.

Privilege makes it easy to acknowledge our controllables when we've had an idea that we've had control all along. Think about someone you know who is at least white, middle- or upper-class, able-bodied, living in the United States, and working with limited medical conditions that affect their well-being. Yeah, they've had their fair share of suffering, and the color of their skin, socioeconomic status, and health outlook (uncontrollables) don't push them further from the starting line for growth and healing. Those with privilege might have an easier time identifying opportunities in their life because they're used to having these opportunities. Those without this may have to work harder, and it's not impossible but effortful at times. I'm putting it lightly here, but you catch my drift.

Everyone has a different starting line, and it's important to account for those things. Those who don't have as much (or any) privilege may struggle to find these opportunities or see how they apply to them. The key is to acknowledge the barriers (we all know our barriers) and to do a deep dive to figure out the opportunities, even if they're small. I like to see sleep as a small opportunity for people to have a little more control over their lives because we all deserve to feel empowered in some way even if society has failed us.

"Kristen, I might have opportunities in life, but I'm stuck thinking about all the barriers, so why even try?" Yes, all these feelings are valid, and this is a black-and-white view. Even more deeply, all feelings are valid but not all behaviors are. You're allowed to feel like shit about all this stuff. The key isn't to make that feeling go away or pretend it doesn't exist. If we did that, it would be invalidating and not fun. Accepting that you have barriers in life doesn't mean you agree with these barriers. But accepting that does help you acknowledge where to go from here. It gives you a sense of empowerment for even a small second. You can hate every minute of this, but I'm encouraging you to care about your sleep because existing (in general) matters. And if you're fearful of doing this, then do it terrified. Do it angry. Do it frustrated. It's okay to feel this and do something good for yourself. You know what the outcome will be if you don't make a change because you're living it right now. This is the rest of your life if you decide to stay put, which is also valid if that's your choice.

Everyone I've met has had something to teach me. Everyone. Even if I didn't realize it at the time. And if you're here, it means your presence contributes something to the world. You might read some tips in this book and be like, "Okay, this doesn't really apply." Fair, but what parts of it can apply? We're not looking for perfection here but gradual, small progress in the right direction.

If we collectively enhance our sleep as a society, I think we will experience less overall pain and be able to be present to live our lives to the fullest. We won't need to cancel life events to sleep more. We can show up and parent our children easier. We can listen to the elderly lady tell us her life story on the bus because she has nobody to talk to. We can attend that women's march to advocate for our reproductive rights. We can take time to vote and sign policies to promote helpful LGBTQIA+ and sex education in schools. We can learn more about the lives of minorities and how to help them as white people. We can attend our daughter's wedding and support her to the fullest. We can allow ourselves to grieve the loss of our baby for the first time because we aren't so sleep-deprived. You see where I'm going with this.

The relationship we have with ourselves affects all others. If you're a little more rested, you might have more pep in your step, and you can help someone in need. Or, most importantly, you can find and be open to receiving the help *you* need to reduce your pain.

Chapter 3

INSOMNIA MYTH-
BUSTING TIME

There's a lot of stuff in the depths of the internet. You can search and get a response for anything. Ask any question your heart desires. If you're an expert in something, you'll probably read some of these answers online and think, *I can't believe this information is out there, damn.* Maybe you know some of it is bullshit and some of it is fact. A layperson might not realize that, so it's important to dispel any myths about these topics. Information can be helpful but also harmful, so it's important to use discernment and double-check your resources to be sure.

It's crucial to do your research, as well as consult with people who have in-depth training about insomnia. I see the client as the expert on their life experience, and I'm the expert in clinical psychology and insomnia. I have never been in my client's shoes, so I have limited information about their lived experience, what feelings they have, or their perspective on certain topics. They haven't completed all the training we have as clinical psychologists to understand the nuances of diagnostic categories, how to rule out diagnoses, and how certain diagnoses influence treatment outcomes. The best part is that we are a highly effective team when we stick together because we have different viewpoints on the same situation, which helps people get better. That's why therapeutic rapport is so important. On top of it, I'm not an academic researcher; I'm a clinician. So, I rely on our sleep research heroes to provide us with this information so I can do my job effectively. There are plenty of experts; you just need the right ones in your corner.

Another reason why the doctor-client relationship is so important is the potential to expand perspectives on both ends. Have you ever had a conversation with someone and left with a different perspective, or you became curious about things in a different way than when you originally started? That's kind of like insomnia treatment, and even you reading this book. You might read some stuff and not realize how it can change your perspective. This is one of the most valuable parts of learning, connecting, and reflecting.

There's a lot of talk about self-diagnosing and how people can treat their disorders. I appreciate people taking stock in learning more about their symptoms and doing their research, and honestly, they should. Finding reputable, peer-reviewed sources helps us learn the most about our symptoms. Reading from various sources (not just one article or one journal) that have reliable and valid measures is important, even if the research contradicts your original viewpoint. That's the cool thing about research. You might have an idea about what's happening in your mind or body, and after a lot of research you might find that it's something else. Or you'll find that your original thought was correct. Either way, you have more information now and know how to proceed. Your therapist studies these things for a living, and getting their take might help because they train for years to filter out certain symptoms and diagnoses.

Quite frankly, I love when my clients find a relatable video and show me, saying, "*This* is what I mean when I say I experience insomnia." It shows what they experience in real-time when they can't sleep at night. It gives me such good information about how the person experiences the world. However, this isn't the same as diagnosing. Having collateral information is helpful, and psychologists use this when they conduct assessments, but it's not the same as looking at all the other nuances and seeing how this particular symptom relates to a client's presenting concern. It can be damaging to self-diagnose and call it a day without getting the perspective of a professional because there are so many symptoms that overlap. It's the same with insomnia. Like we discussed earlier, there are over seventy sleep disorders, and difficulty falling asleep is a symptom that may be part of many of these diagnoses or even unrelated diagnoses.

The internet is littered with information about sleep. There are many insomnia myths that the general public assumes to be true. My colleagues and I are like, "Really? They actually wrote that in a blog?" Some myths are obviously false, some not so much. Let's get you up to speed on the major myths and see how we can use the right information to guide our sleep health in helpful ways.

Myth One: You Need Eight Hours of Sleep

Let's start with the heavy hitter.

There are several nuances here. We don't *need* eight hours of sleep per night; this is a *recommended average* number based on normal, healthy functioning adults. The actual recommendation we clinicians use is an hourly *range* rather than one specific number and varies based on age.

Many sources, including the National Sleep Foundation and the Academy of Sleep Medicine, suggest a range of seven to nine hours for young adults and seven to eight hours for older adults to maintain their overall health.[139, 140] Countries like Canada, Australia, and New Zealand don't have a blanket number; they also consider factors that impact sleep duration, such as activity level.[141, 142, 143] The more sedentary you are, the less sleep you might need, which makes sense. If we are sitting all day long, our body isn't using as much energy. And sleep is for restorative purposes rather than relaxation. Our body isn't going to sleep more than it needs to.

You might be the type that functions well on about six to six and a half hours of sleep per night. Some people function even better on ten hours of sleep. And, I notice that if I work out more, my sleep need increases. I think Canada has the right idea here. Some people have a genetic predisposition for shorter sleep.[144] I've learned that this genetic predisposition is rare, so you'll want to check with your doctor to ensure an accurate diagnosis.

The quality of our sleep matters more than the hourly requirement. Striving for more sleep isn't better. It might make you feel like you're doing something good for your body, but in my opinion, it's more important to get six hours of quality sleep than ten hours of broken sleep with frequent awakenings that cause anxiety and stress. While

---

139 Consensus Conference Panel, Non-participating Observers, and American Academy of Sleep Medicine Staff. (2015). Recommended amount of sleep for a healthy adult: A joint consensus statement of the American Academy of Sleep Medicine and Sleep Research Society. *Journal of Clinical Sleep Medicine, 11*(6), 591-592.

140 See footnote 83.

141 New Zealand Ministry of Health. (2017). *Sit Less, move more, sleep well: Active play guidelines for under-fives.* https://www.health.govt.nz/system/files/documents/publications/active-play-guidelines-under-fives-may17.docx.

142 Okely, A. D., Ghersi, D., Hesketh, K. D., Santos, R., Loughran, S. P., Cliff, E. P., Shilton, T., Grant, D., Jones,R. A., Stanley, R. M., Sherring, J., Hinkley, T., Trost, S. G., McHugh, C., Eckermann, S., Thorpe, K., Waters, K., Olds, T. S., Mackey, T. ... and Tremblay, M. S. (2017). A collaborative approach to adopting/adapting guidelines - The Australian 24-hour movement guidelines for the early years (birth to 5 years): An integration of physical activity, sedentary behavior, and sleep. *BMC Public Health, 17*(Suppl 5), 869.

143 Chaput, J. P., Dutil, C., & Sampasa-Kanyinga, H. (2018). Sleeping hours: what is the ideal number and how does age impact this?. *Nature and Science of Sleep, 10,* 421-430.

144 He, Y., Jones, C. R., Fujiki, N., Xu, Y., Guo, B., Holder, Jr., J. L., Rossner, M. J., Nishino, S., and Fu, Y. (2009). The transcriptional repressor DEC2 regulates sleep length in mammals. *Science, 325*(5942), 866-870.

we need more research in this area, there is a loose association between too much sleep and higher mortality rates.[145]

So, I can tell myself, "Let me try to get nine hours of sleep to fit in," and I'll wake up super groggy and fall asleep later the next day because I got more sleep than I needed. I have to base it on my body's expectations and unique needs. More isn't necessarily better. However, sometimes our bodies need more sleep, which is based on a few other factors, like activity level, stress, or health-related factors. If you're running a marathon, then your body will need more recovery time and sleep because muscles repair themselves overnight, too. So the blanket "eight hours" doesn't apply to everyone, and if we blindly accept this as a fact, it can push us further away from achieving quality sleep.

The TLDR: the amount of sleep we need *generally* depends on age, sleep drive (e.g., activity level), and sex assigned at birth. The amount of sleep we actually receive depends on this plus our race, medications, medical conditions, psychological concerns, stress, bed window, and more. Some sources even say eight hours is more than enough sleep for normal, healthy functioning adults.[146] Regardless, genetic factors may explain the differences in sleep needs, although intentionally restricting our sleep throughout our life is not healthy.[147]

---

145 Cappuccio, F. C., D'Elia, L., Strazzullo, P., and Miller, M. A. (2010). Sleep duration and all-cause mortality: A systematic review and meta-analysis of prospective studies. *Sleep, 33*(5), 585-592. https://pubmed.ncbi.nlm.nih.gov/20469800/.

146 Tune, G. S. (1968). Sleep and wakefulness in normal human adults. *British Medical Journal, 2*(5600), 269-271.

147 See footnote 142.

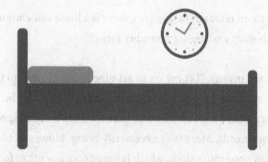

HOW MUCH SLEEP DO WE REALLY NEED ?

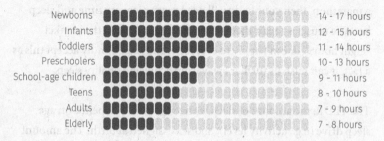

Newborns	14 - 17 hours
Infants	12 - 15 hours
Toddlers	11 - 14 hours
Preschoolers	10 - 13 hours
School-age children	9 - 11 hours
Teens	8 - 10 hours
Adults	7 - 9 hours
Elderly	7 - 8 hours

These sleep ranges also depend on our age. The National Sleep
Foundation suggests that newborns need fourteen to seventeen
hours, infants need twelve to fifteen, toddlers need eleven to fourteen,
preschoolers need ten to thirteen, school-aged children need nine
to eleven, teenagers need eight to ten, adults need seven to nine, and
older adults need seven to eight.[148] I know you're wondering how they
came up with these ranges because I wondered the same thing. The
National Sleep Foundation employed a panel of sleep experts to figure
this out. The panel reviewed 277 studies that explored major sleep
variables such as number of overnight awakenings, how long people
slept, sleep efficiency, and sleep latency, and looked at other variables

148 Hirshkowitz, M., Whiton, K., Albert, S. M., Alessi, C. Bruni, O., DonCarlos, L., Hazen, N., Herman, J.,
      Adams Hillard, P. J., Katz, E. S., Kheirandish-Gozal, L., Neubauer, D. N., O'Donnell, A. E., Ohayon,
      M., Peever, J., Rawding, R., Sachdeva, R. C., Setters, B., Vitiello, M. V., and Ware, J. C. (2015).
      National Sleep Foundation's updated sleep duration recommendations: Final report. *Sleep Health,
      1*(4), 233–243.

that help with sleep health.[149] They came up with these ranges based on data from these studies and their expert opinions. But there is more to sleep than the hourly recommended range.

The Nuances

I'd like to think that these ranges can apply to everyone, but I wonder about other variables that are out of our control, such as disability status, race, ethnicity, chronic pain, socioeconomic status, immigrant status, medical issues, and more. Most scientific studies discuss the extraneous variables they account for, but I imagine that it's impossible to account for everything. This is why it's important to use these ranges as a guide and then see how they apply to our lives with our unique experiences (a.k.a. why most people see me for insomnia treatment because it's individualized).

Chronic Pain and Medical Conditions

A lot affects the amount of sleep we can achieve.

Think about how you sleep when you're sick. When we have the flu we might have more frequent awakenings, wake up feeling exhausted, or feel we need even more sleep because of our symptoms. This may be someone's everyday experience living with chronic pain or a medical issue. They're tossing and turning at night, unable to get comfortable. Once they do, they fall asleep and it's tough to want to get out of bed because their body is begging for more sleep. This person may not

149 Ohayon, M., Wickwire, E.M., Hirshkowitz, M., Albert, S. M., Avidan, A., Daly, F. J., Dauvilliers, Y., Ferri, R., Fung, C., Gozal, D., Hazen, N., Krystal, A., Lichstein, K., Mallampalli, M., Plazzi, G., Rawding, R., Scheer, F. A., Somers, V., and Vitiello, M. V. (2017). National Sleep Foundation's sleep quality recommendations: First report. *Sleep Health, 3*(1):6–19.

want to get up and want to "bed lounge" instead because they are in so much pain. It makes sense from a human standpoint, and this chronic pain experience puts a wrench in the idea of eight hours of sleep. This person might need more sleep because they've experienced ten awakenings overnight, or they might need less because they slept through the entire night, but the pain makes them think they want to stay in bed longer.

In reality, staying in bed longer doesn't cure the pain and causes them to feel like they have less functionality as a human. So they might say to themselves, "Damn, I slept eight hours. I should be good," when their body needs more. On the other hand, they might wake up and say, "Damn, I need more sleep," when their body truly needs movement to get going. This is why I hesitate *only* to look at the numbers rather than the sleep quality. Some studies suggest the quantity of sleep is related to medical conditions or health-related symptoms.[150] We might have to change our perspective and relationship with sleep if we have uncontrollable conditions, and we may need more or less sleep. It's more about listening to our bodies and seeing how we feel relative to other days. Taking data is valuable and helpful in situations like these.

How do we take data? Well, Chapter 7 will give you a full visual!

Chronic pain is only one example of how our medical conditions affect sleep time. We know that overall health and sleep health are related and impact one another.[151] Poor sleep is associated

---

150 Moore, P. J., Adler, N. E., Williams, D. R., and Jackson, J. S. (2002). Socioeconomic status and health: the role of sleep. *Psychosomatic Medicine, 64*(2), 337-344.

151 Grandner, M. A. (2014). Addressing sleep disturbances: An opportunity to prevent cardiometabolic disease? *International Review of Psychiatry, 26*(2), 155-76.

with inflammation,[152] weight gain,[153] mortality,[154] diabetes,[155] and cardiovascular issues.[156] You can imagine that sleep time may be affected based on the side effects of these medical conditions. For example, those who experience physical and emotional discomfort from their body shape and weight may experience difficulty getting comfortable at night. They might need more pillows or provisions to reduce the pain points in their bodies. Those with diabetes or cardiovascular issues may need medications that have side effects for poor sleep. They may need to administer medications at certain times, which may wake them up or disturb their sleep cycle. They might need to wear uncomfortable monitors, even when they sleep.

Socioeconomic Status, Education, and Race

Another factor is socioeconomic status, which not everyone has control over. It's unusual that we jump from poverty to making seven figures a year within a short time. So, we can assume that socioeconomic status may be a more stable, uncontrollable factor relating to sleep. What shocked me was that many early research studies about sleep didn't consider race or ethnicity. I even think about how health researchers define race and ethnicity today and how these classifications may not fully capture differences among groups.[157]

---

152 Grandner, M. A., Sands-Lincoln, M. R., Pak, V. M., and Garland, S. N. (2013). Sleep duration, cardiovascular disease, and proinflammatory biomarkers. *Nature and Science of Sleep, 5,* 93-107.

153 Patel, S. R. (2009). Reduced sleep as an obesity risk factor. *Obesity Reviews, 10*(Suppl 2), 61-68.

154 Gallicchio, L., and Kalesan, B. (2009). Sleep duration and mortality: A systematic review and meta-analysis. *Journal of Sleep Research, 18*(2), 148-158.

155 Morselli, L. L., Guyon, A., and Spiegel, K. (2012). Sleep and metabolic function. *Pflügers Archiv - European Journal of Physiology, 463,* 139-160.

156 Grandner, M. A., Chakravorty, S., Perlis, M. L., Oliver, L., and Gurubhagavatula, I. (2014). Habitual sleep duration associated with self-reported and objectively determined cardiometabolic risk factors. *Sleep Medicine, 15*(1),42-50.

157 Kaplan, J. B. "The quality of data on "race" and "ethnicity": Implications for health researchers, policy makers, and practitioners." *Race and Social Problems 6,* no. 3 (2014): 214-236.

Race is traditionally considered a biological marker linked with physical characteristics, whereas ethnicity alludes to cultural expression and identification with certain social groups. But then there's variability within racial groups themselves, which leads me to believe that simply using "race" as a factor reduces it to a biological definition without meaningfully capturing someone's lived experience related to racial discrimination, which affects health outcomes, stress, and sleep. I think there should be more studies about how racial discrimination affects sleep, but I digress.

Think about the stress of someone living under the poverty line. They may not be as concerned with sleep, but more so about their next meal. The eight-hour rule might not even be realistic for them because they are searching for a place to simply exist because they don't have stable housing. We refer to this as limited sleep opportunity. They might get a few good nights of sleep in a house, then not have this stable housing for the rest of the week or month. Someone who experiences this may think, *My sleep varies from night to night. I can't even count on eight hours, let alone a safe place to sleep.* What's more realistic is thinking about the small, day-to-day opportunities in which they can achieve even a few hours of sleep rather than trying to fit them in this eight-hour box with no awakenings. The eight-hour idea isn't inclusive and doesn't shed light on the broad human experience.

One study suggested sleep disparity experiences are influenced by socioeconomic status, race, and education. Keep in mind as you read studies, in general, that they all have limitations. I encourage people to read the articles cited in the footnotes after reading my (brief) summary. Anyway, this 2010 study by Patel and his colleagues was pretty incredible. They examined income, education, and employment and sleep attainment among 9,714 randomly selected people through a self-report questionnaire in Philadelphia. They noted that those who identified as Latinx and African American were more likely to experience poor sleep when compared to whites. Those who experienced low income or unemployment were more likely to experience poor sleep. The more education someone had, the better their sleep outcomes were reported. Interestingly, African American and Latinx populations living in poverty had the worst sleep outcomes, but whites living under the poverty line had the highest likelihood of poor sleep outcomes. However, as whole groups, African Americans and Latinos had poorer sleep quality and quantity when compared to whites. Those who had at least a college degree were 50 percent less likely to experience poor sleep.[158]

What?! As you can see, looking at your recommended age range and hourly requirement isn't even enough; we have to account for these subtle differences, and we are only hitting the tip of the iceberg. The human experience extends beyond education and socioeconomic status. It's unclear whether race contributes to poor sleep or indirect features relating to the lived experience for certain marginalized groups affect sleep outcomes. If I can take a guess, I think it might be a combination of both.

Another study suggested that health disparities exist even when we control for education and income, suggesting that people of color more commonly experience cardiovascular issues, asthma, and diabetes,[159] which we know may impact sleep health. Also, the neighborhoods we live in affect our well-being (i.e., perception of safety, experience of discrimination, exposure to noise and toxins, or access to healthy food). And who decides what happens within these neighborhoods and how they are structured? Well, society. If we look at sleep, we also have to look at public health. If we look at public

158 Patel, N. P., Grandner, M. A., Xie, D, Branas, C. B., and Gooneratne, N. (2010). "Sleep disparity" in the population: Poor sleep quality is strongly associated with poverty and ethnicity. *BMC Public Health, 10,* 475.

159 Grandner, M. A., Williams, N. J., Knutson, K. L., Roberts, D., and Jean-Louis, G. (2016). Sleep disparity, race/ethnicity, and socioeconomic position. *Sleep Medicine, 18,* 7-18.

health, we have to look at people's day-to-day experiences and how this impacts their well-being. If we change the sleep world, we'd have to account for these things outside of our control.

Isn't there more about race and sleep? Yep. There's more than I can ever cover in this book, but here's a sneak peek. Some research suggests that Black individuals sleep less and less efficiently as compared to other races,[160] especially when compared to their white counterparts.[161] Researchers also suggest that African Americans, on average, may obtain less slow-wave sleep and make up for this in lighter sleep stages, which suggests that their sleep is less restorative.[162] And to top it all off, minorities in general may experience lower quality sleep when compared to whites.[163]

What accounts for this? Well, I don't know, absolutely everything? ;) The Black experience is vast and dynamic, from experiencing systematic racism in society to experiencing microaggressions to leaving a store with nothing in hand and wondering if someone's thinking you're stealing something because of the color of your skin. Or rushing to work because you need to pay your bills and getting pulled over and fearing for your life. Or not being able to sleep at night because you're wondering if you'll get selected for the new position among a group of white applicants. Or being the only person of color in your neighborhood and wondering how other people view you.

---

160 Mezick, E. J., Matthews, K. A., Hall, M., Strollo Jr., P. J., Buysse, D. J., Kamarck, T. W., Owens, J. F., and Reis, S. E. (2008). Influence of race and socioeconomic status on sleep: Pittsburgh sleep SCORE project. *Psychosomatic Medicine, 70*(4), 410–416.

161 Ruiter, M. E., DeCoster, J., Jacobs, L., and Lichstein, K. L. (2011). Normal sleep in African-Americans and Caucasian-Americans: A meta-analysis. *Sleep Medicine, 12*(3), 209–214.

162 See footnote 160.

163 Jean-Louis, G., Kripke, D. F., Ancoli-Israel, S., Klauber, M. R., Sepulveda, R. S. (2000). Sleep duration, illumination, and activity patterns in a population sample: Effects of gender and ethnicity. *Biological Psychiatry, 47*(10), 921–927.

These are extremely small examples of what might keep people up at night or hinder them from getting the sleep they need. I write this knowing I will never understand exactly what it's like, even if I take hundreds of training sessions and talk to a million people. It's not how it works, and I know this is only the tip of the iceberg. So if you're thinking about more shitty things you experience as a person of color living in the world right now, add all of that in right here: ____. I shortened the line for writing purposes, but we know it can take up an entire book.

So, if you think the "eight-hour" recommendation doesn't apply to you, that's okay. It doesn't apply to everyone because we all have unique experiences. Is it helpful for our health to be in the seven-to-nine range (if you're an adult)? Of course. But this may not be possible with your life experiences. So what do we do about this? The key is to not be so hard on yourself if you can't achieve quality sleep in this way and try to manage the stressors outside of your sleep health. And, if those stressors aren't controllable, we validate our experiences and try to view them differently without taking away the fact that they are difficult, painful, and unfortunate.

Myth Two: You Can Catch Up on Sleep

The short answer: eh, it depends.

I know this may seem like a buzzkill for some of you reading this, but it's true. People will ask me, "Can't I just catch up on sleep on the weekends?" I mean, technically, yes, but does it do what you think it's going to do? Not really. Our body needs sustainable, consistent sleep to achieve all of the important things that happen overnight. As we've discussed earlier, sleep can help with releasing hormones, forming memories, cell and tissue repair, and regulating emotions, and it helps you feel rested and energetic.[164] When we don't have enough time to do this, our bodies may not be able to restore what they need overnight.

We call these missed sleep opportunities "sleep debt." It's the amount of sleep you need versus the amount of sleep you actually achieve. It's a cumulative calculation, so going to sleep an hour later or waking up an hour earlier each day adds to your overall sleep debt. By the end of the week, you might have a sleep debt of five hours. Think about sleeping your ideal seven hours plus five hours. That's twelve hours of sleep that you'd need to "catch up" on. Even if you can sleep twelve hours, it doesn't do what you think it does. Your body is just exhausted at this point.

"But I feel so rested on the weekend after I sleep twelve hours." That can be true. What's also true is that your body was most likely struggling Monday through Thursday on four hours of sleep with you working a full-time job, dating, taking care of your kid, going out for happy hour with friends, and trying to maintain a 3.5 GPA. Oh, on top of bingeing your new favorite show and avoiding burnout from your job. Perhaps you're also trying to train your dog not to bark at the mailman. Small stressor, but big annoyance. Enough to cause frustration and hinder your parasympathetic nervous system from being the main character.

Researchers have found that compensating for sleep on the weekends doesn't restore our capacities in the same way that consistent,

---

164 MedlinePlus. (2017). *Healthy sleep*. U.S. National Library of Medicine. https://medlineplus.gov/
      healthysleep.html.

consolidated daily sleep does.[165] Some studies also suggest that cisgender women are more likely to experience sleep debt when compared to cisgender men. This same study also suggested that those who are low-income, less active, and partnered with children are more likely to experience severe sleep debt.[166] So, the American dream of getting married and having kids also reduces our sleep quality? Just kidding, but really: kids can be wild and wreck our sleep! And we love them anyway.

This exhaustion is similar to driving under the influence of alcohol. What?! Lack of sleep is similar to being drunk? Yep, without the hangover, but the effects might be worse. We also know that short sleep and sleep deprivation are associated with higher mortality rates.[167] For example, the Centers for Disease Control (CDC) suggests that being awake for over eighteen hours is similar to having a blood alcohol content (BAC) of .05 percent.[168]

Even if we think about this daily, our bodies tell us that we aren't functioning properly off short sleep. We talked about the detrimental effects of sleep deprivation, sleep inefficiency, and poor sleep quality in an earlier chapter, and that all applies here.

---

165 Leger, D., Jean-Baptiste, R., Collin, O., Sauvet, F., and Faraut, B. (2020). Napping and weekend catchup sleep do not fully compensate for high rates of sleep debt and short sleep at a population level (in a representative nationwide sample of 12,637 adults). *Sleep Medicine, 74,* 278–288.

166 See footnote 164.

167 Ma, Q. Q., Yao, Q., Lin, L., Chen, G., and Yu, J. (2016). Sleep duration and total cancer mortality: A meta-analysis of prospective studies. *Sleep Medicine, 27–28,* 39–44.

168 Williamson, A. M., and Feyer, A. (2000). Moderate sleep deprivation produces impairments in cognitive and motor performance equivalent to legally prescribed levels of alcohol intoxication. *Occupational and Environmental Medicine, 57*(10), 649–55.

Naps

What about naps? Well. It depends on your sleep goals and sleep opportunities. Some people want that consolidated sleep at night with limited awakenings. In that case, we advise against napping. However, if you are exhausted and know that a nap will be rejuvenating, we suggest a thirty-minute nap to ensure you are rested and ready to take on the next activity for your day. A short nap can help restore your mental capacities and working memory for a few hours. Napping truly varies from person to person. Some doctors will suggest naps for some people but not others after doing a sleep assessment. Individualized sleep recommendations are important, so seeing your doctor on this one might be a good starting point.

Then, there's another elephant in the room. I'm going to start naming these elephants; maybe we can name this one Mia. Anyway, some people may not have adequate sleep opportunities. They may work a job or two and they're a caregiver for a parent. Maybe they live in a low-income neighborhood and they're up a little later because they're not sure if their partner will come home at night. They might feel fearful about what might happen during sleep, so they distract themselves with another job so they don't have to be home. They finally get home at midnight and have to wake up at five o'clock for their first job. So they have a sleep opportunity of five hours, which is lower than the recommended daily average for adults. They may lie in bed awake due to anxiety, or they might have some space to think about the day. Then, they wake up and do it all over again. Sleep debt increases in this situation, and this person may or may not be able to even "catch up" on sleep the next day. If they had napping opportunities, I would suggest this person take them because their opportunities for sleep are limited. Their circadian rhythm may be screaming at them, but at least they are getting some sleep. Sometimes we have to choose between two shitty decisions: nap and have a lower sleep drive at night or stay awake, be exhausted, and have a higher likelihood of accidents or mistakes.

We know that napping can be helpful for shift workers and those prone to driving long distances.[169] I like to call these naps "safety naps." They ensure your safety and are needed to prevent accidents. I think about working moms who, after coming home exhausted, have to take care of their kids. They may doze off on the couch for a little nap and then they can make dinner and engage with their kids. Without that nap they probably would be irritable and have less patience when helping their kids with homework. Think about if this mom had to get in the car to drive her kid to basketball practice. Yikes, that wouldn't be so safe, right? Naps might help.

But Wait, There's More

Can sleeping in on the weekends fully restore our bodies? When we compare it to consistent daily sleep, not really. It's just not the same. It can be restorative, but it doesn't hit like a solid seven or eight hours of quality daily sleep. But that's not to say it's not helpful.

One study compared mortality rates among people with short sleep during the week with more sleep on the weekend, and those people didn't differ much from those who had consistent sleep.[170] In this same study, people who didn't sleep much on the weekdays or weekends had increased mortality rates. So if we're not getting enough sleep overall, we know it's not helpful for our health. However, if catching

---

169 Faraut, B., Andrillon, T., Vecchierini, M. F., and Leger, D. (2017). Napping: a public health issue. From epidemiological to laboratory studies. *Sleep Medicine Reviews, 35*, 85-100.

170 Åkerstedt, T., Ghilotti, F., Grotta, A., Zhao, H., Adami, H., Trolle-Lagerros, Y., and Bellocco, R. (2019). Sleep duration and mortality–Does weekend sleep matter? *Journal of Sleep Research, 28*(1), e12712.

up on sleep on the weekends is your only opportunity for now, it's not terrible. It just isn't ideal.

Another study described that this pattern of weekend recovery sleep doesn't reverse the metabolic dysregulation that happens when we lose sleep during the week.[171] Big yikes. My generalized psychologist answer here is: *it depends*, but I always like to err on the side of caution and try to help people get quality daily sleep while addressing the limitations of sleep opportunities for certain populations. If you're staying awake to watch television or scroll social media, I'd say that some of this is within your control and we can be more curious about how this keeps us up later than expected. However, if factors in your life prevent you from having an opportunity to sleep, that's a little different. You might try to sleep when you can. It's likely something outside of your control.

Myth Three: No Overnight Awakenings Means I'm Sleeping Well

Have you heard of people saying they sleep through the entire night and don't wake up at all? Or maybe you remember a time in your life when you used to sleep through the entire night. Well, that is possible. I sometimes see sleep data that suggests people aren't aware of their awakenings overnight or they are aware and they are short-lived, so they aren't designated as awakenings, even though that technically counts. Another thing to consider is that we aren't the best historians when it comes to our sleep and remembering our awakenings. Can you remember how many times you woke up overnight last Tuesday?

---

171 See footnote 124.

It's similar to remembering exactly what you ate for breakfast a few days ago. You may have experienced awakenings overnight but don't remember them because they were short-lived or were too exhausted or groggy to categorize them as an awakening.

The short answer is: most people experience a few short-lived awakenings overnight.[172] For adults, I usually look at their overall presenting concern, including stress, chronic pain, medical conditions, circadian rhythm, sleep drive, and environmental factors that may impact awakenings. I do this to see if these awakenings make sense based on their conditions or if it's insomnia (or a combination of both). Someone with chronic pain may wake up more than someone without this condition. The same goes for the elderly population. We sleep less as we age and experience more frequent awakenings overnight. Something to look forward to! (sarcasm)

Yeah, another buzzkill. But it doesn't have to be. Let's chat about the reasons for these awakenings and why it's okay to see them as somewhat normal. A study from 2010 mentioned that about one-third of people experience overnight awakenings, and these awakenings were more likely to be associated with psychiatric disorders and organic diseases.[173] In my practice, I've only encountered a few clients who slept throughout the entire night with no awakenings at all. Then again, take this with a grain of salt because most people see me for treatment for this exact reason because they can't sleep through the night.

---

172 DerSarkissian, C. (2022). *Waking up in the middle of the night.* WebMD. https://www.webmd.com/sleep-disorders/stay-asleep.

173 Ohayon, M. M. (2008). Nocturnal awakenings and comorbid disorders in the American general population. *Journal of Psychiatric Research, 43*(1), 48-54.

What Is a Nighttime Awakening?

For simplicity reasons, let's categorize these nighttime awakenings as observable and non-observable. We might have several non-observable awakenings. It's helpful to explain the non-observable ones through the lens of sleep architecture. When our body is powering through the sleep cycles (e.g., REM, N1, N2, and N3), it experiences more REM sleep toward the latter end of the night as the body prepares for its final awakening. Sounds so serious, right? Well, it kind of is. When controlling for all other variables, your body may naturally awaken when you're in a lighter stage of sleep. You're so close to being awake, and your body may think it's show time.

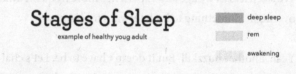

Stages of Sleep
example of healthy youg adult

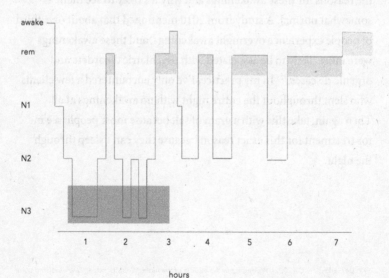

hours

Other things account for nighttime awakenings, which I'll get to. But the observable awakenings, well, you know what that feels like. You wake up in the middle of the night, check the clock, and it's two in the morning. You've been awake for thirty minutes now. Wide. Awake. "I think I fell asleep around ten o'clock, so why is my body waking up all of a sudden?" You're lying in bed, remembering the horrific date you went on earlier. The gal you met online wasn't exactly who she said she was. She did not look like her picture, so you feel catfished. Not to say she wasn't wearing makeup; she was a completely different person. "How could I be so dumb? Am I that easy to trick?" The date went well but you felt uncomfortable because you didn't know how to say it. You didn't know how to say, "Hey, are you who you say you are?" You work through all the red flags, including the ones you overlooked, and you're lying in a pool of shame in your bed. The shame is everywhere, contaminating your pillows and your idea of going back to sleep.

This sort of awakening is observable and may be because of anxiety or stress. Maybe this was already on your mind before bed, so it's likely your brain is still working through this scenario, which is why it's essential to have a solid bedtime routine if your schedule allows. These observable awakenings may be more within our control (compared to non-observable ones), and we can use strategies to reduce these experiences. However, it depends on the person and their unique situation. More on this later.

Same-Time Nocturnal Awakenings

"What if I'm waking up at the same time every night? It's like my body loves to wake up at three in the morning and waste my time." This is a bizarre feeling. Each night you put your head on the pillow, knowing that three o'clock will greet you before you know it. And *bam*! No alarm, no external noise. You wake up for seemingly no reason, no meeting, no purpose. It's dark and cold in your room and you're lying there. Your body simply wakes up and you struggle to get back to sleep. This observable awakening feels frustrating. "I've tried everything; why is this happening?" There might be a few reasons for this.

You'll want to check with your doctor before anything because it can be an underlying medical condition or an undiagnosed sleep disorder. If both of these check out and there are no glaring issues, I usually (generally) blame circadian rhythm or sleep cycle. This varies for everyone, but these are typically the culprits. As we discussed earlier, circadian rhythm is the twenty-four-hour cycle that regulates our sleep-wake patterns, and sleep cycle is the way our bodies move through different stages of sleep.

Sometimes our body's circadian rhythm isn't aligned with our bed window preference. This means that we *want* to be a morning person, or the person who falls asleep early, or the person who can stay awake until one in the morning and sleep until eight o'clock, but maybe our body isn't designed that way. This means our chronotype (a.k.a. our body's natural sleep preference) isn't aligned with our sleep expectations. We can work to alter this in some way, but it's best to do this under supervision (a.k.a. with your sleep specialist or doctor).

With this in mind, our body may be pushing to honor its natural chronotype. It's basically like, "Come on, girl; let's get this day rolling," and you're like, "Okay, but it's quite literally three in the morning." Your body might be trying to tell you something. Maybe you've already slept about eight or nine hours and don't need any more sleep (even though you want it). You might also feel tired, but that's not a reason to go back to sleep after sleeping a full nine hours. Your body might naturally wake up at this time and be ready to start the day because of your underlying chronotype. But there may also be other reasons you wake up consistently throughout the night.

Factors That Impact Nocturnal Awakenings

I know you're thinking, *What else can there possibly be? How will I handle all these factors that impact my nightly awakenings?* Don't worry. I have a few ideas about this. Some of these factors are within our control and some aren't. For the ones we can't control, we may have to adjust our expectations around sleep. It's almost like expecting things to happen and not shaming yourself for them rather than forcing them not to happen and failing in the process.

Meals

Although there needs to be further investigation in this area, some researchers suggest that large meals close to bedtime may influence quality sleep and nighttime awakenings.[174] One study described that university students who ate a meal within three hours of their identified bedtime were more likely to experience disrupted sleep (e.g., overnight awakenings) compared to their non-meal counterparts.[175] Another study described that meals close to bedtime (e.g., within one hour of intended bedtime) were associated with longer sleep duration but more fragmented sleep.[176]

Who doesn't like to munch a bit before bed? I know I do, but I also notice I have a few more awakenings overnight and I wake up feeling a little off. However, I know people who eat a full meal before bed

---

174 Kinsey, A.W., and Ormsbee, M. J. (2015). The health impact of nighttime eating: Old and new perspectives. *Nutrients, 7*(4), 2648–2662.

175 Chung, N., Bin, Y. S., Cistulli, P., and Chow, C. M. (2020). Does the proximity of meals to bedtime influence the sleep of young adults? A cross-sectional survey of university students. *International Journal of Environmental Research and Public Health, 17*(8), 2677.

176 Iao, S., Shedden, K., Jansen, E. C., O'Brien, L. M., Chervin, R. D., Knutson, K. L., and Dunietz, G. L. (2020). 0221 Late meals, sleep duration, and sleep fragmentation: Findings from the American Time Use Survey. *Sleep, 43*(Suppl 1), A86.

and wake up feeling fine. This is one of those factors that you'll have to see what works for your body. And being honest with yourself is important. Maybe you enjoy eating before bed, but you know it isn't good for you. Both of these thoughts can be true, and we can avoid meals during certain times if it helps our sleep.

We know that some meals shorten our sleep onset, which helps us fall asleep faster, but most studies suggest wrapping up any eating at least three hours before bedtime.[177] The type of meal matters, too. Meals with a low glycemic index are likely to be a better choice than a heaping bowl of pasta before bedtime. I love pasta, so I hurt my own feelings as I wrote this. However, there are some studies out there that suggest high-glycemic meals may help with total sleep time and sleep efficiency, but they didn't mention anything about awakenings.[178] It's important to consider your medical conditions here. For example, doctors may encourage some patients to eat a small meal before bedtime to maintain blood sugar levels.

But, why though?

Our bodies mostly focus on all the processes we discussed earlier (e.g., cell and tissue repair, memory consolidation, energy restoration, metabolism, and temperature regulation). A primary focus on digestion is another (potentially) avoidable burden to add to the list. If our body normally does all these other things overnight, and suddenly it has to digest a huge plate of lasagna, it might lead to more awakenings. Of course, we know some carbohydrates help us feel a little drowsy and may aid in falling asleep. That's not to say it helps with other aspects of sleep, such as awakenings.

---

177 Afaghi, A., O'Connor, H., and Chow, C. M. (2007). High-glycemic-index carbohydrate meals shorten sleep onset. *The American Journal of Clinical Nutrition 85*(2), 426–430.

178 Vlahoyiannis, A., Aphamis, G., Andreou, E., Samoutis, G., Sakkas, G. K., and Giannaki, C. D. (2018). Effects of high vs. low glycemic index of post-exercise meals on sleep and exercise performance: A randomized, double-blind, counterbalanced polysomnographic study. *Nutrients, 10*(11), 1795.

As you can tell, the research is all over the place, but it truly depends on what you're looking for. If you're more concerned about awakenings, safe to say you should avoid meals close to bedtime (if you can swing this). If not, meals close to bedtime might not be so bad if awakenings aren't on your list of woes. When in doubt, eat a small snack with a balanced protein-to-carb ratio rather than a four-course meal before bed, and try to make this meal at least three hours before you fall asleep.[179]

Medications

Oh boy. This section can be the entire book because certain medications truly affect our sleep (in helpful and unhelpful ways). I'm not a prescriber by any means—I mostly conduct psychological assessments, consultations, and evidence-based therapy. But we have to be well-versed on medication side effects to know how to help our clients navigate these issues if/when they voice concerns about them. I know that medications can affect our sleep-wake cycles, overnight awakenings, time it takes to fall asleep, and more. A prescriber knows more than me about medication-related things, so it's important to always discuss your concerns with them because we know this book isn't a replacement for medical advice. However, knowledge is power, so let's chat about them. We can talk for hours about medications and how they impact sleep, so I'll touch on the most common ones here.

Certain medications are prescribed for certain sleep issues. It's important to consider your initial diagnosis and what your doctor says. The medications discussed below may be indicated for acute insomnia, chronic insomnia, or something other than sleep issues. Some

179 Madzima, T. A., Panton, L. B., Fretti, S. K., Kinsey, A. W., and Ormsbee, M. J. (2014). Night-time consumption of protein or carbohydrate results in increased morning resting energy expenditure in active college-aged men. *British Journal of Nutrition, 111*(1), 71–77.

are over-the-counter (OTC) medications; others are prescription medications. I'll give you an idea of what they're used for and how they affect sleep.

OTC Sleep Aids

Some sleep aids are available over the counter, a.k.a. you can purchase them without a prescription. Most of them include diphenhydramine, which is the active ingredient in a popular antihistamine that's pink. Regardless, this antihistamine has a natural sedative effect. The other class of other-the-counter drugs includes doxylamine, the primary ingredient in Unisom. Doxylamine is an antihistamine normally used to relieve seasonal allergies (and, in some cases, the common cold). The natural effect of these drugs: they make you drowsy. If you're drowsy, guess what, you have a higher likelihood of falling asleep.

But how effective are these drugs? Well, it depends on what you use them for. The active ingredient in them must be FDA-approved, unlike dietary supplements like exogenous melatonin. If you're jet-lagged and need to get back on a sleep cycle (a.k.a. acute insomnia), these OTCs are recommended if you aren't into waiting it out. On the other hand, if you've struggled with poor sleep and insomnia for years, chronic use of these OTCs may not be most effective. It may impact your awakenings (or lack thereof). Research suggests that diphenhydramine lacks clinical evidence that supports its efficacy.[180, 181] It's hard to say how helpful this is for our sleep. Other studies suggest it only reduces sleep onset by an average of eight minutes.[182]

---

180 Culpepper, L., and Wingertzahn, M. A. (2015). Over-the-counter agents for the treatment of occasional disturbed sleep or transient insomnia: a systematic review of efficacy and safety. *The Primary Care Companion for CNS Disorders, 17*(6), 26162.

181 See footnote 179.

182 Sateia, M. J., Buysse, D. J., Krystal, A. D., Neubauer, D. N., and Heald, J. L. (2017). Clinical practice guideline for the pharmacologic treatment of chronic insomnia in adults: An American Academy of Sleep Medicine clinical practice guideline. *Journal of Clinical Sleep Medicine, 13*(2), 307-349.

Is eight minutes worth the next-day hangover effect? That's not to say it can't be helpful for some people. Again, it depends on what you use these for because it's super effective for allergic reactions.

You might notice that when you take an OTC medication for sleep, you fall asleep *hard*. Meaning, you notice the internal cues of sleepiness and you end up passing out quickly. But what happens to our sleep architecture? I'm glad you asked [insert smirk emoji here]. Research suggests that certain medications can affect our sleep architecture.[183] As you recall, sleep architecture is a fancy term for how our sleep is organized into stages. It's separated into REM and non-REM. Certain stages of sleep are important for certain biological and cognitive processes. If we aren't flowing through the stages of sleep (e.g., wake, N1, N2, N3, and REM), it's questionable whether our body is doing what it needs to do. So even if we sleep through the entire night with no awakenings, I'm doubtful of their helpfulness for our sleep health in the long term.

Just so you know, I'm not against the use of these OTC medications. I mostly like to educate folks to ensure using these aligns with their sleep goals. We know that long-term use of OTC medications for chronic insomnia may not be the most effective option, but if you use these and wake up feeling great and have no issues, then I'm not going to be the one to tell you to stop! But maybe your doctor can shed light on how it may affect your unique concerns.

---

183 Kirsch, D. (2022). *Stages and architecture of normal sleep*. UpToDate. https://www.medilib.ir/uptodate/show/7710.

Benzodiazepines

So, this drug class is somewhat of a touchy subject and primarily used to treat anxiety; it is otherwise known as alprazolam or diazepam. When studying for my licensure exam, we had to memorize some of these medications, and I remember these because of the "pam" or "lam" at the end. Anyway, they slow down messages from the brain and have a sedative effect. If we peel back the onion, benzodiazepines affect our neurotransmitters, namely gamma-aminobutyric acid (GABA), by reducing the activity of our nerves. This drug is mostly prescribed for those who experience panic attacks (at least that's what I notice in my practice). These drugs have a high propensity for dependence. It's not that many people intentionally seek this drug out, but they may notice a physical dependence effect if they are prescribed it for something like anxiety.

My take on benzodiazepines is twofold. It slows our cognitive functions so that we can feel relaxed. This is helpful if someone is experiencing a panic attack. However, we can use strategies to achieve this effect naturally. It may not happen as quickly and we might experience increased fear or frustration, but it's something we can technically work on. It also depends on the person; some people may have organic issues that inhibit them from working on their emotional regulation skills, such as a traumatic brain injury or certain psychiatric diagnoses. All the strategies in the world might not work for that person, and medication like this might enhance their quality of their life.

Secondly, the benefit of this drug can also be a detriment. Think about what happens when our brain function slows down. We might not feel as aware or able to make correlations or connections with the world around us. We might feel light and relaxed, but our problems didn't spontaneously go away. We might wake up the next morning still feeling the weight of our issues. We just took a little break from them. However, I notice that some of my clients report feeling even worse the next day because they didn't have the faculties to handle their issues while taking this medication. Basically, if we take a benzo, our thoughts and fears go into a black box, and then we open that black box when we wake up the next morning. Some people may need some space from their thoughts, but I think other strategies may not have such big side effects.

Research shows that benzodiazepines may decrease the amount of time we hang out in non-REM stage 2 sleep (a.k.a. light sleep).[184, 185] However, benzodiazepines may also spark parasomnias, which are odd sleep behaviors that occur overnight (e.g., abnormal dreams, sleep eating, sleep driving, nightmares, or calling people on the phone in our sleep). If we're experiencing these parasomnias, we likely aren't experiencing quality sleep. So, this is technically an awakening, but maybe one that we're not consciously aware of.

Most people report helpful effects from this drug but at a cost. When discontinuing this medication, some people may experience rebound insomnia,[186] which is basically a fancy word for sleep that is dramatically worse than before starting the drug. This may spark more awakenings overnight. So, in terms of a harm-reduction approach, benzodiazepines may not be the most useful drug to specifically target enhancing sleep quality or helping our body flow through the sleep stages in a natural healthy way (yes, that includes normal awakenings overnight).

184 Proctor, A., and Bianchi, M. T. (2012). Clinical pharmacology in sleep medicine. *International Scholarly Research Network ISRN Pharmacology, 2012.*

185 Ribeiro de Mendonça, F. M., Ribeiro de Mendonça, G. P. R., Souza, L. C., Galvão, L. P., Paiva, H. S., de Azevedo Marques Périco, C., Torales, J., Ventriglio, A., Castaldelli-Maia, J. M., and Martins Silva, A. S. (2022). Benzodiazepines and sleep architecture: A systematic review. *CNS & Neurological Disorders-Drug Targets, 22*(2), 172-179.

186 Roehrs, T., and Roth, T. (2022). *The effects of medications on sleep quality and sleep architecture.* UpToDate. https://medilib.ir/uptodate/show/7704.

Antidepressants

There's a wide range of antidepressant classifications and types. You may have heard of selective serotonin reuptake inhibitors (SSRIs), tricyclic antidepressants (TCAs), or monoamine oxidase inhibitors (MAOIs). Maybe you've heard of none of these, and that's okay because we're here to navigate this together. In grad school, I jokingly called MAOIs mai tais (like the cocktail) because I couldn't figure out what they were until a professor gently reminded me it was a class of antidepressants. Swerve, we don't need to remember embarrassing moments. Anyway, I'll extend that gentle reminder: you're here to learn, not to know everything. Chin up!

Some people are prescribed antidepressants for the exact reason you're thinking: they're depressed. These antidepressants have side effects on our sleep, especially when it comes to overnight awakenings. Research suggests that some antidepressants have a natural effect of decreasing sleep latency (a.k.a. the time it takes us to fall asleep) and reducing our awakenings, which are mostly the tricyclic antidepressants. However! (Buckle up for this one.) The mai tais appear to increase our nightly awakenings and reduce our sleep time. Who would have thought! Additionally, SSRIs are similar to TCAs; they tend to increase our nightly awakenings.[187]

What about the relationship between antidepressants and sleep architecture? You already knew I was going here. I know we aren't supposed to play favorites, but I do. I'm obsessed with the idea of sleep architecture and how cool our body is that it even has a structure like this (insert gif of me hugging my sleep architecture tightly). Wow, I didn't realize I needed to get that out.

---

187 See footnote 185.

Most antidepressants aren't good for our REM sleep because it slows the onset of our REM cycle. Consequently, we may get less REM sleep than we need. I know you want to know the worst and the best ones, and poor MAOIs are at it again, with the worst in class for sleep architecture. So, it's unknown how many more awakenings one might have because of antidepressants, but it's likely to affect them in some sense. What antidepressants *are* good for: reducing symptoms of depression. You might have to make a choice here. Taking antidepressants might help your quality of life even if your sleep suffers. If it were up to me, I'd take the medication and reduce my expectations for sleep. Knowledge is power, so if you know this is you, you might be a little easier on yourself when it comes to your sleep if taking these medications. It's always helpful to chat with your doctor about making a decision about medications, too.

Dietary Supplements: Exogenous Melatonin

Exogenous means it's the synthetic version, not the version made in our bodies.

I know there are some melatonin cheerleaders and haters out there. I'm somewhere in the middle on this one, but I like to defer to the research. Melatonin is naturally produced in our bodies; it doesn't directly cause sleepiness, but it starts an orchestrated event that leads to us becoming more chill. It's the conductor in a music show—the instruments play because the conductor is there. Exogenous melatonin means we are taking a synthetic version of melatonin in pill form. Our body recognizes it as melatonin, but we don't have to create it ourselves.

Our natural melatonin helps with the timing of our circadian rhythm. Our brains start to produce it once the sun goes down or it notices darkness.[188] In a perfect world if you controlled all confounding variables (yes, everything ranging from mood disturbances to financial health to privilege to Pete Davidson's looks and how they affect your concentration), melatonin would naturally secrete around the same time each day if we woke up at the same time each day. We know how crazy this sounds, and how it isn't ideal to be able to control all these events *and* wake up at the same time each day. You might be able to achieve waking up around the same time each day, which is better than nothing. It's somewhat within your control. It's something that I try to say is a good replacement for the idea of exogenous melatonin because we already have it. We just have to create an environment that helps it show up better.

What's the tea on exogenous melatonin? It's a dietary supplement, meaning the FDA does not regulate it. It doesn't mean it can't be helpful for some people, but I like to know what's in the bottle. Since the FDA doesn't regulate it, we are unsure of how much melatonin is in the bottle compared to what the label says, and it may contain other ingredients that aren't purely melatonin. I'm sure places create synthetic melatonin that test their supply, but it's notable to mention that the FDA doesn't approve of it specifically for insomnia yet. Researchers in a study from 2017 examined thirty commercial melatonin supplements and found that melatonin content varied about 10 percent in about 71 percent of these supplements, and 26 percent contained serotonin.[189] Additional serotonin can be harmful to those already taking SSRIs (antidepressants). I'm not sure if you've heard of serotonin syndrome, it's a serious condition with a bunch of physical side effects, and some can be fatal.[190] Of course, side

---

188 See footnote 58.

189 Erland, L. A. E., and Saxena, P. K. (2017). Melatonin natural health products and supplements: Presence of serotonin and significant variability of melatonin content. *Journal of Clinical Sleep Medicine, 13*(2), 275–281.

190 West Valley Medical Center. *4 reasons to be cautious about melatonin.* https://westvalleymedctr.com/blog/entry/4-reasons-to-be-cautious-about-melatonin.

effects depend on your overall physiology, medical conditions, and medications. I know we view serotonin as the happy neurotransmitter, and it has a functional role in melatonin secretion, but it's important to look at this from a harm-reduction approach. Just because we want more serotonin doesn't mean it will actually be helpful or effective for us as it relates to sleep.

Melatonin may have meaningful effects for those experiencing circadian rhythm disorders.[191] Some research suggests that melatonin is helpful for delayed sleep phase syndrome (DSPS) and regulating sleep-wake patterns for people experiencing blindness.[192] Remember, our sleep-wake patterns (regulated by circadian rhythm) are regulated by exposure to light and consistency. Initially, I thought this sort of makes sense with blindness, depending on the severity of their condition. But I learned that the brain still processes light even without vision,[193] so it's kind of a weird correlation. Oh, and DSPS is technically a circadian sleep disorder. It's when the body's internal sleep-wake cycle is weakened or misaligned with their preferred bed window. People with this condition might have trouble making it to work or school the next day due to falling asleep late.

Melatonin may also help with short-term relief of jet lag[194, 195] or assist shift workers[196] because their schedule is likely unpredictable at times. If it's constantly changing, we can assume that melatonin production may be inhibited in some way. In fact, this study suggests

---

191 van Maanen, A., Meijer, A. M., Smits, M. G., van der Heijden, K. B., and Oort, F. J. (2017). Effects of melatonin and bright light treatment in childhood chronic sleep onset insomnia with late melatonin onset: A randomized controlled study. *Sleep, 40*(2).

192 Auld, F., Maschauer, E. L., Morrison, I., Skene, D. J., Riha, R. L. (2017). Evidence for the efficacy of melatonin in the treatment of primary adult sleep disorders. *Sleep Medicine Reviews, 34*, 10–22.

193 See footnote 189.

194 Herxheimer, A. (2014). Jet lag. *BMJ Clinical Evidence, 2014*, 2303.

195 Choy, M., and Salbu, R. L. (2011). Jet lag: Current and potential therapies. *Pharmacy & Therapeutics, 36*(4), 221–231.

196 Sharkey, K. M., Fogg, L. F., and Eastman, C. I. (2001). Effects of melatonin administration on daytime sleep after simulated night shift work. *Journal of Sleep Research, 10*(3), 181–192.

that melatonin secretion is suppressed for those who engage in shift work.[197] However, their circadian rhythm is likely misaligned regardless, so melatonin doesn't cure the problem; it just aids in helping shift workers fall asleep at odd times, such as when the sun is still up.[198]

Think about your body naturally producing melatonin and then you take exogenous melatonin on top of this. Your body is probably like, "Damn, we really out here flowing through a sea of melatonin tonight, huh? We must be exhausted." You fall asleep, but guess what? The melatonin that you took earlier is pushed through your body and metabolized. What happens when it fully metabolizes? Your body sees this as less melatonin, so it thinks it's ready to wake up. Guess what? Then you might have an awakening.

How do these awakenings happen? We're not fully sure, but I'll briefly tell you about my thoughts on the underlying mechanisms. Again, this is brief and my whole point is to assess whether melatonin is the best or most effective strategy for every person. For some people, yes. For all people? No.

The half-life of fast-acting melatonin is between twenty and forty minutes. Let's back up. A half-life is the way that we figure out how long it takes for a medication to be fully processed and excreted from the body. That means that half of the melatonin is still in your body for about thirty minutes, and melatonin is at its peak within an hour. But we experience, I don't know, four to six sleep cycles that are ninety minutes each, so the exogenous melatonin will technically run out and

---

197 Wei, T., Li, C., Heng, Y., Gao, X., Zhang, G., Wang, H., Zhao, X., Meng, Z., Zhang, Y., and Hou, H. (2020). Association between night-shift work and level of melatonin: Systematic review and meta-analysis. *Sleep Medicine, 75*, 502–509.

198 See footnote 195.

not be in our bodies anymore. Your body sees this lack of melatonin as a signal.

What about extended-release melatonin? Sure, this can be helpful for people with certain conditions, as discussed above. You might wake up exhausted and groggy, but I wonder about your actual sleep architecture. Is your body flowing through the sleep cycles naturally when taking a synthetic substance? If we're taking a substance to help keep us asleep, we wake up exhausted but don't have to "deal" with anything else overnight. I'm sure people are stressed and simply want to sleep as a coping mechanism, but it's important to remember the overall function of sleep. Sleep is for restoration, not for relaxation or a tool to reduce stress. The point is to feel more refreshed in the morning. Food for thought.

Of the research available, some suggest melatonin may increase our nightly awakenings[199] while others suggest it may reduce these awakenings.[200] It's hard to tell because of the mixed evidence and research in this area. If you think about testing anything, you first have to know that what you're studying is reliable. Melatonin supplements aren't regulated, so it's hard to know how much is in each bottle. Even when researchers control this, they still denote that melatonin isn't a reliable supplement for insomnia or sleep symptoms. There also isn't technically a recommended dose of melatonin, but some researchers suggest taking the lowest possible dose so your body sees it exactly as natural melatonin (in terms of how it's secreted).[201] It's just a free-for-all out there.

---

199 See footnote 190.

200 Zhang, O., Gao, F., Zhang, S., Sun, W., and Li, Z. (2019). Prophylactic use of exogenous melatonin and melatonin receptor agonists to improve sleep and delirium in the intensive care units: A systematic review and meta-analysis of randomized controlled trials. *Sleep and Breathing, 23*(4), 1059-1070.

201 Vural, E. M. S., van Munster, B. C., and de Rooij, S. E. (2014). Optimal dosages for melatonin supplementation therapy in older adults: a systematic review of current literature. *Drugs & Aging, 31*(6), 441-451.

At the end of the day, I am a consumer of research and a clinical
psychologist by trade. We like to look at the data and the evidence, and
it isn't all there for melatonin right now. It's promising, but we need
more trials and more regulation of these supplements to say for sure.
That said, your doctor will know more about what's right for you, and
you might know what's right for you, if the evidence is mixed. I like
to do experiments sometimes after talking to my doctor. I might tell
them, "Hey, I'm gonna give this a whirl and take some data. I'm going
to take melatonin for a few days, stop for a few days, then look at all my
awakenings." My doctor usually gives me some good advice of what to
look out for and how to take data in helpful ways.

Hormones

When I think of hormones I think of puberty. Oh gosh, do you
remember when you went through puberty? I don't want to remember
it, actually. I remember bumping into things more often because
my hips were getting wider. I was so upset back then. If I could talk
to younger Kristen now, I'd say, "This is one of your body parts that
you'll grow to love. Be patient." Our bodies are in constant flux. We
don't know who we are; we're figuring out our preferences for partners
and where we belong in the world. We're suggestible and want to fit in,
desperately trying to make it to class without embarrassing ourselves
or being the topic of conversation. We walk into a room, and we
think everyone is looking at us (we call this the spotlight effect). It's
tumultuous. I can't imagine being a young person right now. Things
were easier when I was younger because we had flip phones and no
way to screenshot text messages. It seemed like there were no rules.

When we're younger, we sleep more due to secreting human growth
hormones. An early study from 1989 noted that growth hormones
were secreted during sleep, reaching a peak about an hour after sleep

onset.[202] Researchers suggest this is especially prominent for newborns and babies because, well, they're growing exponentially. We believe this hormone is secreted at night, and guess what? They do sleep more. As we age, we need less of this hormone because we're already grown up, but it's still needed for building muscle or recovering after exercising. We just don't need so much of it as we did when we were babies. Anyway, this hormone affects our sleep duration because we sleep less as we age.

Okay, where's the juicy stuff? Other hormones affect our sleep. We know that cisgender women are more likely to experience sleep disturbances than cisgender men. I'd love to know more about nonbinary individuals here because we need more data points rather than the binary. There's some data to suggest transgender and nonbinary individuals may also experience poor sleep.[203]

Then there's menopause. Ah, hot flashes and discomfort. Something to look forward to, right? Menopause usually means hormonal changes will take place, meaning women tend to secrete less estrogen. These changes happen even years before the onset of menopause (also known as perimenopause). We talked about temperature earlier, so I'm sure you know where I'm going with this. Hot flashes cause a spike in temperature, causing some women to experience more awakenings overnight.

---

202 Takahashi, Y., Kipnis, D. M., and Daughaday, W. H. (1968). Growth hormone secretion during sleep. *The Journal of Clinical Investigation, 47*(9), 2079–2090.

203 Harry-Hernandez, S., Reisner, S. L., Schrimshaw, E. W., Radix, A., Mallick, R., Callander, D., Suarez, L., Dubin, S., Khan, A., and Duncan, D. T. (2020). Gender dysphoria, mental health, and poor sleep health among transgender and gender nonbinary individuals: A qualitative study in New York City. *Transgender Health, 5*(1), 59–68.

Cortisol

The stress hormone. This description says it all. When we're stressed, it can be difficult to sleep. Well, there's more to it than that. Researchers believe one of the functions of sleep is cortisol management, and it plays a role in maintaining your sleep cycle. When we have an increase in cortisol, our body becomes more alert, reducing melatonin secretion. Toward the end of the day, cortisol levels decrease and melatonin increases. They miss each other at the party every time but for good reasons.

Biology story time (shortened version). Cortisol is most notably associated with the "fight or flight" response, but not in the way you're thinking. Cortisol doesn't trigger this; adrenaline does. Our body identifies a stressor or trigger (e.g., something you're experiencing in real time, maybe a trigger to a past event, or even an intense intrusive thought) and it releases adrenaline so you can be on top of your game. Then, cortisol is released, helping your body by releasing glucose from your liver. This glucose helps us fuel whatever we're ready to do because of this threat (i.e., our body thinks it may need energy to fight or run). It's pretty wild how this happens. However, the function of cortisol extends beyond our stress response and initiating wakefulness as part of our sleep-wake cycle. It helps regulate your metabolism and blood pressure and suppress inflammation.

Elevated cortisol levels happen for various reasons. Most of the time it's for good reasons. Maybe we got scared or became anxious about something. Maybe something is stressing us out. It makes sense and that's why our bodies are designed this way. However, chronic cortisol elevation might affect not only our health but also our sleep.

Elevated cortisol levels may inhibit us from sleeping at night. It helps the body know it's time to stay awake, so this may not be so helpful at night. Think about anything that causes stress or anxiety. You might have an uptick in cortisol even if you watch a scary video on your phone. You aren't experiencing it in real life, but your body doesn't see it that way. It's responding to a stimulus, even if it's on your phone. So you can only imagine if you saw a huge bear in real life. Your body would be like, *Yep, pump out the cortisol!*

That's why we focus on relaxation strategies in insomnia treatment. We try to figure out how to engage the parasympathetic nervous system (relaxation response) rather than the sympathetic nervous system (stress response). I'm sure there are outliers here, but most of the time we don't experience these two simultaneously. You finally lie in bed and maybe your stress response is the main character and your relaxation response is a supporting cast member. We want to switch these roles to feel relaxed and ready for sleep. If cortisol is bumping through our body, it's unlikely that this relaxation comes naturally.

How Lifestyle Habits Affect Awakenings

These are some of the controllables in our life but within reason. Sometimes we have to choose between two pretty shitty decisions. Do I drink caffeine to get through the day and struggle to fall asleep later, or remain groggy throughout the day and fall asleep easier? Sometimes these choices aren't actually choices; they're modes of survival. If you rely on a paycheck, and this paycheck is based on your productivity, the answer is clear. In this case, we have to accept our sleep health and the fact that this is what we're capable of right now. This can help with those nightly awakenings.

I think it would be easy for anyone to say, "I mean, just get up at the same time every day, don't worry about anything, and be happy." Well, if that was the solution, I wouldn't be writing this book, and you wouldn't be internally screaming at yourself for your sleep issues. Also, this comes from a place of privilege. Some people can operate this way and can reduce their stressors because of various reasons. If you had a solution for your stress, you would have acted on it by now. It's just not that easy.

I like to view our sleep health in a specific way. Yes, there are strategies to help enhance your sleep health. Can you act on these right now? Perhaps. Maybe you won't wake up at the same time every day, but maybe you can expect certain things on certain days. You can find consistency in unique or creative ways. If you can't do this, you have to have some grace with yourself and focus on what you *can* control. This might be how you talk to yourself after a rough night or how you treat yourself after you can't fall asleep. The frustration is valid, and you're also a human being. Human beings also need compassion. So, I'm saying that these lifestyle habits might not be fully achievable for you right now, and that's okay. But take note of how you're treating yourself in the process because this matters.

Have you heard of the studies about plants and how talking to them might help them grow faster? Well, we're not sure if there's evidence to support this, but we do know talking to humans in empathetic, compassionate ways helps fuel connection and well-being. When we direct this compassion inward, we validate our experiences and help to acknowledge that we may be suffering, and other people in our situation would feel similarly (a.k.a. self-compassion). When we remove this self-compassion, it's hard for us to acknowledge that our feelings are valid. All feelings are valid, but not all behaviors are, so if you can act on these lifestyle habits but don't feel like it, that's something to be curious about.

These lifestyle habits can range from exercise to food intake, so I'm going to touch on the most important ones (in my opinion).

There are more out there, but these are the ones I notice affecting awakenings the most.

Exercise, Caffeine, and Naps

Good ol' exercise. If we're sedentary, it's likely that our body may not need to rest as much during sleep as it would if we were active. If we are sitting around all day doing nothing, we can't expect to have ten hours of sleep with no awakenings unless there's an underlying medical condition. If we work, exercise, walk to and from rooms all day, keep our minds occupied, and haven't sat for more than twenty minutes at a time, yeah, we're likely to need some more sleep. Your body has more to restore.

Exercise has beneficial effects on your health all around, especially for sleep. Researchers suggest those who exercise experience less WASO (wake after sleep onset, a.k.a. nightly awakenings) than those who do not exercise at all.[204, 205] The same goes for caffeine. Those who limit caffeine intake, especially in the latter half of the day (if they have a traditional bed window), are less likely to experience awakenings and have better sleep efficiency.[206]

Similarly, those who engage in long naps throughout the day are less likely to need more sleep at night, resulting in either more awakenings or an earlier final awakening.[207] We've talked about naps

---

204 Stutz, J., Eiholzer, R., and Spengler, C. M. (2019). Effects of evening exercise on sleep in healthy participants: A systematic review and meta-analysis. *Sports Medicine, 49*(2), 269-287.

205 Edinger, J. D., Morey, M. C., Sullivan, R. J., Higginbotham, M. B., Marsh, G. R., Dailey, D. S., and McCall, W. V. (1993). Aerobic fitness, acute exercise and sleep in older men. *Sleep, 16*(4), 351-359.

206 Lunsford-Avery, J. R., Kollins, S. H., Kansagra, S., Wang, K. W., and Engelhard, M. M. (2022). Impact of daily caffeine intake and timing on electroencephalogram-measured sleep in adolescents. *Journal of Clinical Sleep Medicine, 18*(3), 877-884.

207 Monk, T. H., Buysse, D. J., Carrier, J., Billy, B. D., and Rose, L. R. (2001). Effects of afternoon "siesta" naps on sleep, alertness, performance, and circadian rhythms in the elderly. *Sleep, 24*(6), 680-687.

before, but here's a small refresher and some new information. The
timing, duration, and frequency of these naps are notable. Those
who are chronic nappers and nap later in the day are more likely to
experience awakenings throughout the night and have trouble falling
asleep compared to those who either nap earlier or don't nap at all.[208]
Sometimes these naps are important because they help people stay
alert, especially if they drive vehicles, operate machinery, or engage in
shift work for a living. Naps can be useful to enhance performance if
one is feeling extremely sleepy.[209]

Those who enjoy napping or sleeping in segments: if it's not broken,
don't fix it. If it's working for you, great! You don't have to put yourself
in the "consolidated sleep" box if that's unrealistic for your unique
life circumstances.

Naps and caffeine aren't bad things. I see them as useful tools when
used for specific reasons. It depends on your unique goals and
circumstances. If these cause issues, try to change them. If you can't
change them, change how hard you are on yourself. If you *can* change
them, and it sucks, welcome to the shitshow. Reducing caffeine and
naps can be difficult. I limit caffeine about once a year to test my body
(is this normal?). I sometimes last a few months, other times a few
weeks. It all depends on what's going on in my life. I notice that during
periods of intense stress, I drink coffee more. Everyone's different.

Sometimes it's about prioritizing movement, which is related to our
sleep drive. Sleep drive is the body's biological need for sleep. If you
run five miles, your body probably needs more rest than if you sat
around. We chatted earlier about how sleep drive is similar to our

208 Mograss, M., Abi-Jaoude, J., Frimpong, E., Chalati, D., Moretto, U., Tarelli, L., Lim, A., and Dang-Vu,
     T. T. (2022). The effects of napping on night time sleep in healthy young adults. *Journal of Sleep
     Research, 31*(5), e13578.

209 Signal, T. L., Gander, P. H., Anderson, H., and Brash, S. (2009). Scheduled napping as a
     countermeasure to sleepiness in air traffic controllers. *Journal of Sleep Research, 18*(1), 11-19.

hunger drive; once we eat a meal, our hunger drive decreases. Once we wake up from a full night of sleep, our need for sleep decreases. Over the course of the day, this sleep drive increases, then we have those internal cues of sleepiness, then boom! We hit the pillow and pass out.

Sleep drive is increased by exercise, limited caffeine, and avoiding naps. If we do all of these things, we will likely have more consolidated sleep at night. We won't wake up as much because our body genuinely needs rest. Avoiding these things and increasing exercise might not be realistic for some. In that case, you need to meet your body where it is. If you're napping, drinking caffeinated beverages, and not exercising, your body may not need as much sleep as you think. Yes, you might still wake up feeling unrested, but your sleep drive is relatively low. You might have trouble falling asleep or staying asleep. So, if you're going to engage in these lifestyle habits, it's not a bad thing. But what *is* bad is doing these things and expecting your body to fall asleep when you want it to. This goes back to our expectations about sleep. If our sleep drive is low, we might have a difficult time getting to sleep. Expecting this is helpful, though, so we don't shame ourselves into sleep.

Stress Management, Screentime, and Buffer Time

Other habits to consider as they relate to nightly awakenings include avoiding screen time at night (or in bed), using stress management tools, and buffering time before bed.

It depends on what we're searching for on our phones, but screen time may impact our ability to feel fully "chill" upon going to sleep, and we might wake up thinking about things we've searched for. Or not. Everyone is different.

Having strategies to reduce stress also helps us prime our minds and bodies for sleep, as well as having an adequate buffer time before bed. We know that even anticipating a stressful event can impact our awakenings and sleep efficiency.[210] If you can't get rid of the stressor (most of the time you can't because if you could have, you would have by now), you have to figure out how to manage your stress response, while also validating the fact that this is, in fact, a stressful situation. So many nuances here, but they are important.

If we allow ourselves to feel sad or angry about a situation and then figure out how to somewhat accept it, it helps us come to terms with the fact that we might not have control over it. We experience slight relief because we're thinking about it differently and holding space for our emotions while acknowledging that this stressor cannot be fixed. You don't have to agree with the stressor, but accepting that there's no solution and that you can't fix it also helps you know where to go from there. I'm not saying to disregard your feelings, but regard them with full force and allow yourself to take some space from it, just for the sake of your sleep. You can always revisit it the next day. I ask myself, "Will this matter in a year?" If the answer is no or maybe, I use this as an indication to revisit it tomorrow. If the answer is yes but I can't do anything about it now, I also revisit it tomorrow. Perspective sometimes helps.

A buffer time is a time you set aside to prepare to relax and engage before bed. It's almost like priming a wall before you paint it. You'll get the color on there, but it's likely to look better with primer. Our sleep benefits from certain tools that we use beforehand, and these are some of them. I usually dim the lights during this time and put on relaxing music. I play the same playlist every night and find myself

---

210 Beck, J., Loretz, E., and Rasch, B. (2022). Stress dynamically reduces sleep depth: Temporal proximity to the stressor is crucial. *Cerebral Cortex, 2022.*

almost priming my brain for sleep with this consistency. Ideally, we do this about an hour before bed. Sometimes we can't, though. I'll provide alternative solutions as you read along.

Okay, so where's the data? Researchers suggest screen time right before bed may influence the time it takes us to go to sleep, how well we sleep, and how many times we wake up throughout the night.[211, 212] Of course, screen time is variable, depending on your age, race, and life circumstances, but researchers say that screen time is overall associated with poorer sleep quality, which may mean more awakenings.[213] Let's also consider the type of screen time. There are clear differences between searching "most horrific things to happen in America right now" and "cute puppies frolicking in a lavender field." We might have feelings and reactions to these that impact our sleep.

The Apprehension

I'll die on this hill: if you have an opportunity to implement these, great; if not, we look at other ways to enhance sleep, even just a little bit.

It doesn't mean you fail at sleep; it means you gotta get creative. Because you are unique, and your situation calls for something different. You might not have much time before bed to just chill or relax. You might need your phone close if someone calls because you're dealing with a family issue. You might also not have many

211 Hysing, M., Pallesen, S., Stormark, K. M., Jakobsen, R., Lundervold, A. J., and Sivertsen, B. (2015). Sleep and use of electronic devices in adolescence: Results from a large population-based study. *BMJ Open, 5*, e006748.

212 Cabré-Riera, A., Torrent, M., Donaire-Gonzalez, D., Vrijheid, M., Cardis, E., and Guxens, M. (2019). Telecommunication devices use, screen time and sleep in adolescents. *Environmental Research, 171*, 341–347.

213 Christensen, M. A., Bettencourt, L., Kaye, L., Moturu, S. T., Nguyen, K. T., Olgin, J. E., Pletcher, M. J., and Marcus, G. M. (2016). Direct measurements of smartphone screen-time: Relationships with demographics and sleep. *PloS One, 11*(11).

stress management tools, or the ones you have aren't feasible at home because you live with a bunch of people. Take these tools, pick them apart, and find a small, related thing that might fit for you. For example, you might not have an entire free hour before bed. But you might have somewhat of a bathroom routine where you brush your teeth, wash your face, and put on lotion. That might take you about five to ten minutes. You can use that five to ten minutes to decompress, do some deep breathing, and be intentional with how you're showing up during this time. You might feel exhausted and cranky; that's okay. We hold space for those emotions while also giving ourselves some TLC.

If you have an opportunity to implement these things but don't want to, let's be curious about how it's impacting your life. Sometimes we have to do things we hate to feel better. You don't have to get rid of the "hate" part; you can allow that to exist and do the thing anyway (oh, the dialect). I remember feeling resistant to implementing certain sleep strategies even though I knew they were in my control. I had to tell myself that I do have a choice in *some* sleep situations. *I don't have many choices in other areas, so if I can make a good choice for my health, this kind of seems like self-care, and I deserve that.*

I sometimes scroll on my phone in bed. I hit snooze. I take naps. I drink caffeine. And sometimes I don't do those things. On the days that I don't, sleep seems to be better. On the days that I do these things, I sometimes wake up more than usual, experience daytime fatigue the next day, or go into a shame spiral of self-loathing because I can't "get it together." The last part is the part that's within my control the most. This is all part of the process. There's always room for improvement and growth, and sometimes that's acknowledging what we don't want to change even if we have the opportunity. If we know that we can put our phones down but don't want to, that's okay. The natural consequence is that you might fall asleep later, but the self-loathing that comes with it can be altered.

Do you hate yourself, or are you filling your needs at the time and it has a consequence that you're not happy with? Are you more upset about your ability to have self-control or your tiredness the next day? Are you upset with your life circumstances that you can't change and want to but can't? These questions help you figure out if it's you, the uncontrollable life circumstances, or your general hesitancy to show up in a way that helps you feel better. Sometimes we want to stay in pain. Not everyone does, but it's something to consider if you're struggling to implement things, even if you want to.

Myth Four: Our Body Gets Used to Less Sleep

Well, this would be convenient, right? If we had to sleep less, we'd have time for more activities. We'd be able to work more, maybe have more fun with friends. It doesn't quite work this way. The hard truth is that you might be good at managing your life on less sleep, but your body doesn't ever get used to it.

It's almost like your manager expects you to complete a bunch of tasks in a limited amount of time. Can you get it done? Probably. Will it be quality work? Not likely. This is kind of how sleep works. If you're only sleeping a few hours per night, your body will take it, but it doesn't restore your functions to their full capacity or potential with less time. In fact, depending on how much sleep you're losing, this can be detrimental to your health. Another buzzkill, I know. But I want you to be informed, okay? Don't hate the messenger (a.k.a. me), but if you do, I'll take it. Just read the rest of this so you know how it'll affect you. :)

A few nights of poor sleep won't hurt us. However, when we chronically deprive ourselves of much-needed sleep, our bodies experience some serious effects. We're less able to make clear decisions, struggle to remember things, and are less creative. Over time, we notice this deprivation is likely to affect our cardiovascular system and metabolism.[214] It can also affect mental health,[215] which we know is closely aligned with our physical health. Our immune systems also suffer,[216] making fighting off infection and disease difficult. We talked earlier about how important our immune system is and how it's our internal army. We want that army to be ready for battle.

As you can tell, our bodies don't adapt to restricted sleep or sleep deprivation over time. Well, you will notice that you are still alive, but your body is struggling to keep it all together. This is especially true for those who are more active. Our bodies need more rest when we exercise, as we discussed earlier. Another point is that you might not be aware that your body is struggling, but it is. Researchers have found that people who restrict their sleep report more stress and inflammation,[217] whereas those who increased their total sleep time by 7 percent report fewer mood disturbances and experience less inflammation.[218]

---

214 See footnote 128.

215 Freeman, D., Sheaves, B., Waite, F., Harvey, A. G., and Harrison, P. J. (2020). Sleep disturbance and psychiatric disorders. *The Lancet Psychiatry, 7*(7), 628–637.

216 See footnote 128.

217 Lorenzetti, M. S., Skicki, J., Craddock, T. J., and Tartar, J. L. (2017). 0084 The psychological and physiological implications of sleep restriction: A comparison of voluntary and experimental sleep restriction groups. *Sleep, 40*(Suppl 1), A32.

218 Famodu, O. A., Montgomery-Downs, H., Thomas, J. M., Gilleland, D. L., Bryner, R. W., and Olfert, M. D. (2017). 0083 Impact of a single week of sleep extension on performance, mood, and nutrition among female college track athletes. *Sleep, 40*(Suppl 1), A32-A32.

I know there are a lot of blogs that provide tips on how to get used to less sleep. I was shocked when I saw this. I was like, *Damn, they're really out here telling people the wrong stuff about sleep.* I was pleasantly surprised, however, when I learned most of these blogs acknowledge that chronic sleep deprivation is bad, and they provide some sleep hygiene tips. I think it's all about sleep opportunities and how we prioritize sleep. If we don't view sleep as an essential function, it's less likely that we will try to create time for it.

That said, quality sleep is better than simply getting those eight hours. If you're sleeping for seven hours with limited awakenings, that's better than ten low-quality hours. Work smarter, not harder, right? So we might try to make those seven hours count instead of striving for more than that. Even if we get ten hours, it might not be so helpful. You might cut out certain substances that are toxic to your body or prepare yourself for rest before you get into bed. We'll talk about some strategies in this book to get you into a place where your body is primed for sleep, even if your bedtime window and opportunity aren't much.

Myth Five: Bed Lounging Will Help You Fall Asleep Faster

This is another one that sounds like it would work out for the best, but most of the time it doesn't help our sleep health. This one has a lot of gray areas because some people can lie in bed and not care that they're falling asleep quickly. But, if you're reading this, you're likely one of those people who hop into bed and your brain starts moving a mile a minute. I'm one of those people, too. I said it a few times and I'll say it again: it all depends on your sleep goals. If you're bed lounging and you don't care and it's not affecting your sleep or your life, keep it goin'! For those who struggle, keep reading.

Think about when you think you have your shit together, so you hop into bed earlier than usual. Sometimes you're exhausted and you pass out quickly, but most of the time you're probably awake longer than usual. "Why, though? I'm in bed earlier, so I should fall asleep earlier so I can get more sleep." Yeah, most people have thought this. But you're doing your body a disservice if you get into bed when you aren't sleepy.

Remember when we chatted before about the difference between internal cues of tiredness versus sleepiness? Let's revisit that. Our body will only sleep if it's sleepy. If we're tired, we may feel exhausted, but our bodies don't need sleep; they need relaxation. And it's okay if this sounds annoying, inconvenient, or aggravating. Most of us want to "catch up" on sleep or reestablish a good bedtime routine by getting into bed early and lounging We sometimes think lounging in bed, or getting into bed earlier, will help us fall asleep quicker. I wish this was the case because it would be the easiest fix for someone with insomnia.

We notice that people who bed lounge or spend excessive time in bed when they aren't tired tend to make a negative association with their bed. Their brains interpret the bed as a place to stay awake rather than fall asleep. When we do things while we're awake in bed, our brains think this is the time to stay awake, think about stressful stuff, fight with our partner, or that it's a place where we are generally uneasy or uncomfortable.

If we aren't sleepy, then we won't sleep. Our body is awake during this time, and it mentally says to itself, "Okay, we're awake. What should we do? Let's think about a bunch of stuff. Oh! Remember when you had that embarrassing moment at work when you fell in front of your work crush, and now they think you're clumsy? Super cute. Or maybe the time that…" And then what happens? You start to feel stuff. Feelings, yep. Probably embarrassment or shame. Thinking about these things doesn't help you fall asleep quicker. It helps you hate yourself more. Then, your brain thinks this happens every time you get into bed when you aren't sleepy. If it happens enough, your brain thinks this happens even when you *are* sleepy. We've associated our bed with negative stuff. Yikes. This is a slippery slope that we should probably avoid. Sometimes that's not possible, but there's a reason why it happens.

Why Does This Happen?

The science behind this is pretty fascinating. Sometimes we associate the bed with worry or frustration, and sometimes it's associated with sleepiness, relaxation, and calmness. This association is called classical conditioning.[219] Do you remember Pavlov and the dog experiment? If not, I'll give you the inside scoop on how this relates to sleep. It might make it easier to implement changes when we know why things happen.

Ivan Pavlov was a psychologist conducting experiments studying digestion and noticed something interesting about how his dogs behaved when presented with food. He noticed they salivated not when they saw or smelt food but when another random cue was associated with the food itself. So the dogs knew they were going to eat but didn't have the direct cue of the food to inform this response.

219 Perlis, M. L., Jungquist, C., Smith, M. T., and Posner, D. (2005). *Cognitive behavioral treatment of insomnia: A session-by-session guide.* (1st ed.). Springer Science & Business Media.

Pavlov originally thought that the dogs were salivating because they saw the researchers in lab coats, and they associated these lab-coated researchers with food. So he discovered a neutral stimulus (lab coats) is associated with an unconditioned stimulus (something that happens automatically, like eating food), even when both are usually unrelated. Not many of us see researchers in lab coats and think, *Yeah, it's time to eat,* but these dogs did. So he did another experiment to make sure. He rang a bell to associate with the food. He'd present the food while ringing the bell, and the dogs began to salivate. Then, he'd ring the bell without the food, and the dogs would still salivate when they heard it. This is called a conditioned response because it was learned and unnatural. This can be generalized to how we associate our beds or bedrooms with sleep (or not).

Your bedroom may be associated with you being alert, anxious, or frustrated rather than sleepy and chill. A bed itself doesn't automatically evoke this response for every person, but it does for some because we've either learned this by accident or were aware that this was happening. If you're wondering what a conditioned response is, ask yourself if most people would react the same way in this situation. For example, when you hear a loud bang, your body flinches. When you smell food, you know this is associated with hunger and eating. Your eyes water when you cut an onion. Pulling your hand away from a hot stove when nobody told you to do so. It's a natural response that didn't require a lot of (or any) prior learning.

Our bed is normally paired with sleepiness, but sometimes it's paired in different ways that aren't so helpful because, well, we're human. Human experiences are complex and becoming more diverse and unique as we discover more about human behavior. Either way, it doesn't take much for our brains to pair the bed and/or bedroom with certain experiences. It also is something we can actively work on changing to get better sleep. More about this is in the last chapter.

How to Fix It

If you're still reading this, you're most likely struggling with being exhausted and sleepy, then lying in bed and feeling awake. You might also be the type who falls asleep so easily on the couch but not the bed. I'm sure you wish this sleepiness from the couch would transfer to the bed. If I had a magic wand...

The key is to notice that this is happening, so take some data about your sleep habits. Most sleep experts suggest getting out of bed if you can't fall asleep in about twenty minutes. This varies from person to person. Sometimes it takes people longer to fall asleep and they may need to lounge in bed a little longer, (say, for thirty minutes). However, this is not generally the case. If you notice yourself awake, you'll want to get out of bed and do a relaxing activity. Cringe! I know. "But if I stay here a little bit longer..." Nope. Your brain is associating lying in bed with wakefulness, anxiety, or some experience other than sleep. Of course, there are some moments when you'll stay in bed awake for longer for other reasons. Maybe you took your medications late, or life is stressful, or you woke up super late, or you're experiencing jet lag. I'm talking about the chronic paired association of the bed with wakefulness over weeks or months.

I can't tell you how many times I tell my partner, "Hey, I'm getting out of bed to get sleepy," and he nods at this point because he gets it. In the beginning he was like, "Wait, you're gonna do what? That sounds counterintuitive," until he read the research and was like, "Oh yeah, this is pretty cool." He also has zero sleep issues despite being in the military. Not sure how that all worked out. Maybe he's God's favorite, or maybe he has good sleep habits that I don't know about. I'll have to do an investigation here.

The take-home point is basic sleep hygiene: only get into bed when
you notice those internal cues of sleepiness (e.g., nodding off, inability
to stay awake, knowing you'd be super drowsy if you got behind
the wheel), only use the bed for sleep and intimacy, and leave your
bedroom when you're experiencing unhelpful behaviors such as lying
in bed awake or anxious. I *only* enter my bedroom if I'm in a calm
state, which I've had to train myself to do over a few years. If not, I
lie on my couch in the same spot to associate it with my relaxation
station. (Criiiiiiinge, I know, but it works. I fought the feeling forever.)
This small step really helped with my insomnia. There might not be an
opportunity to "spend time awake" when you're exhausted and have
to get up early the next day, or if it's the only opportunity you'll have
all week to have a quiet house. I get it. And your body is telling you
something, so we may as well listen. The end goal is that this sleepiness
translates to the bed, and it's easier to fall asleep over time. If this has
happened for a while, it might take a bit for you to see some results.

Chapter 4

JET LAG AND DAYLIGHT SAVING TIME

Jet lag and Daylight Saving Time. Both wreck our natural circadian rhythm, which is our natural sleep-wake cycle. We haven't talked about yet another elephant in the room. It's kind of shocking so make sure you're sitting down. Our circadian rhythms regulate more than our sleep-wake cycle. I know, it's shocking! Circadian rhythms also help regulate temperature, appetite, blood pressure, and hormone levels within a twenty-four-hour cycle.

Experiencing jet lag and changing the clocks for DST will disrupt these natural rhythms. Consequently, we go through a few changes biologically, but we notice the physical and mental changes more. We might be more sluggish, tired, irritable, and maybe even anxious. You'll also notice you might make more mistakes or have low performance at work. It sucks a lot, honestly.

I'm sure you can relate to the struggle of trying to adjust your sleep schedule when you're in a new time zone or desperately trying to fall asleep earlier to avoid the one hour you'll lose from turning your clocks forward. There may be changes for DST in 2023, you'll want to read more about this because it can change your life in many ways.

Jet Lag

If you've ever flown on a plane across a time zone or two, you know the feeling of jet lag. For those who haven't been on a plane, you might experience this while on a road trip. Road trips don't technically count as jet lag, but not everyone has had the ability to fly, so I want to be inclusive here. The difference with a road trip is that you're traveling at a decent speed (e.g., whatever the speed limit is) and you are aware of the time zones changing, and time moves at a familiar speed.

When you hop on a plane, you'll likely be traveling across a few states to (hopefully) have some fun and when your head hits the pillow, you feel off. You can't explain it. You've traveled all day and haven't napped, but you feel like your bedtime isn't your bedtime. Maybe you get those internal cues of sleepiness way earlier than you normally do. Or maybe they're later than expected. Worst-case scenario, you don't notice the sleepiness cues and you're lying in that hotel bed, wondering when you'll fall asleep. Your body clock seems off, and it's probably because, well, it is. Your circadian rhythm is confused.

What Actually Is It?

Jet lag is a temporary or acute sleep issue that happens when we travel across time zones relatively quickly and have issues adjusting to a different schedule.[220] According to the Diagnostic and Statistical Manual of Mental Disorders, Fourth Edition (DSM-IV), it's technically a circadian rhythm disorder. It's a sleep disruption due to

---

220 Arendt, J. (2018). Approaches to the pharmacological management of jet lag. *Drugs, 78*(14), 1419–1431.

altering our natural sleep-wake cycle or when our natural sleep-wake schedule is misaligned with our environment or professional schedule.

It sounds scary, but your circadian rhythm is super adaptable because it's regulated by consistency and exposure to bright light in the morning and less light at night. The consistency piece may be missing when you experience jet lag because you're in a new, maybe unfamiliar place, without the normal things you have at home.

As if flying across time zones at supersonic speed isn't enough, other factors make jet lag worse. These factors are technically things we can alter or manipulate to the best of our abilities to improve our situations. Some of these aren't exactly what you'd expect.

Sleeping Arrangements

This one is pretty obvious. If you're visiting friends or family, you might be sleeping on a couch or in a guest bedroom, and it's not like your usual sleeping arrangement. If you're in a hotel for a work trip, you'll either have your own space or share a space with someone you don't normally sleep with. These sleeping arrangements are inherently different than your home.

You don't have the comfy pillow or blankets that you'd normally have. Maybe this bed has springs that are uncomfortable or dig into your back. Maybe it's too firm or too soft; it's nothing like your mattress at home. Well, what about the opposite? This bed might be more comfortable than your bed at home, with plush pillows and a cooling topper that keeps you cozy at night. Guess what? You'll probably be sleeping better tonight than you do at home. That's a win. Sometimes these arrangements are better when we're away, which helps our jet lag because we're more comfortable.

You might also notice sounds that are way different from your bedroom. Maybe you sleep with a fan or two and now you're at your mom's house and you can hear a pin drop. You can hear all the conversations through the thin walls; you can hear someone scrolling TikTok at three in the morning with no headphones. You know when someone gets up to use the bathroom and if someone's having trouble sleeping. And their trouble sleeping keeps you awake, too. You hear everything.

If it's not the inside of the home that's keeping you awake, it might be sounds from the outside. If you're used to living in a city and traveling to a more suburban or rural place, well, life is different in those parts of the world. You might hear sounds of nature, like birds or animals, or you might not hear any sounds—a departure from what you normally hear in the middle of the night. You might be used to hearing people walking and talking outside at any time. You're well aware that a train comes by at a certain time or people get up for work at weird hours, so you hear them starting their cars.

If you don't have pets, you might travel to a house with cats, dogs, horses, pigs, or maybe even reptiles that freak you out because you've never been that close to an iguana in your life. Animals make noises and have a certain presence, which is different from your pet-less apartment. Pets are curious creatures, so maybe the family dog wants to sleep in your room or in bed with you. Sleeping with a pet when you're not used to having any is a wild experience. They have dreams like we do, and sometimes they make noises we wouldn't expect. My dog sometimes whines in the middle of the night when he's dreaming. I never know what he's dreaming of, but I want to save him if he's running from a bear. Either way, it would be hard for me to sleep with someone else's dog if they whined differently or generally had different habits.

All these environmental factors usually contribute to our sleep time or sleeping patterns when we're in a new place, and this isn't an exhaustive list. These factors may also contribute to sleep loss or increased sleep time, depending on their helpfulness. Comfortable sheets and a cool dark room might help with sleep, but you might not be used to this because your bed feels different. That alone may be a struggle.

Habits

Our habits are usually different when we're away from home. You don't have your typical meals; you don't have access to your snack closet. You might drink more caffeine than usual or eat more dense meals than you're used to because your body needs some energy. You might sleep in more and not have any sort of schedule. It might be difficult to gauge when to get out of bed and what to do throughout the day. If you're on a business trip, you might have a solid schedule that inhibits you from creating a helpful sleep routine. I'm thinking of business trips when people go to seminars or work events and everyone goes out afterward. Before you know it, it's midnight; you're a few drinks in and not tired at all. Good luck getting to sleep tonight because you'll have to do it again the next day.

Routine

Even if you don't have a solid bedtime routine, you're probably doing a few things to gear up for bedtime. Maybe you come home from work, drop off all your stuff, lay your ass on the couch, and binge the latest crime series on Netflix. Maybe you eat dinner, go for a walk, play with your dogs, and then turn all the lights down. Maybe your kids enjoy being outside before going to bed, so you stay outside with them and watch them ride their bikes without training wheels for the first time.

Some of us have solid bedtime routines. At a certain time every night, you might turn all the lights low, remove electronics from your eyes and hands, and engage in more chill activities. You lightly clean your house, pick up some items and put them back in their original place. You close up your kitchen, intending to revisit it in the morning for breakfast. You walk around to the same side of your bed, like you always do, plug your phone in, and get under your covers. The covers are comfy and predictable; you know the feeling of them and how heavy they are. You turn over, lie on the same side you always do, and wake up the next morning.

Well, none of this is possible when you're in a new place. Your bedtime routine may be way different, and that's just the start. What about your other routines? You might have a partner with whom you do certain things throughout the day or evening. If they're not around, you feel lost and might not have the same routine you do at home. It can also be kind of stressful to think about the fact that you don't have all the comforts of your home, and you realize how comforting those things are, even if you complain about your house, routine, or life situation.

Stress

Even if your hotel bed is the most comfortable, expensive one out there, it's still different from your normal sleeping arrangements. That alone may cause stress or anxiety just because of the unknown. The reasons for your travel might also be a source of stress. Maybe you're traveling back to where you grew up, with all the triggers and stark reminders of your past. You meet up with old friends and family and although it's great to catch up, it's a source of pain for you knowing how life has changed over the years. You might be traveling for a wake or funeral, which isn't fun either.

The stress of flying is also another topic to consider. Even if you don't mind flying, there's a process involved here. You have to wake up at a different time than usual, travel to the airport, get through security, take off half of your wardrobe to go through TSA, and be nervous about them checking your bag even though you aren't a drug smuggler. You finally get to your gate and you're hungry. There are no rules at airports, so you eat something random, like a burger at nine in the morning, and then get in line to board. You have carry-on luggage that you hope can fit in the cabin above your seat; if not, you'll have to find another place for it. You see where I'm going with this. There's a lot to consider, and it might not feel like negative stress, but it's still more to think about.

Combating Jet Lag

There are a few ways to reduce the burden of jet lag, and no, it's not to stop flying altogether to avoid the situation. It's mostly focusing on the things you can control or that you can manipulate. I usually start this process a few days before I hop on my flight, and I separate it into three categories. The first is "what I can do before I leave to come home to an easier house," "shit I can pack to make my life easier," and "mimicking the routine at home."

Before Departure

This is one of the most important parts because it's where a lot of your control is. I clean my entire house, down to the sheets, if possible, before I leave. I have no idea the headspace or mood I'll be in when I return, and I don't want life to be more stressful if I have a tough trip. You might have to jump back into work, so you may as well start the week off right with everything already done before you get home. This includes laundry, cleaning, yard work, checking the mail, cleaning out your fridge, taking the trash out—you get where I'm going with this. Flights get delayed and you might be away longer than expected, so I try to plan for any and all possibilities. I almost expect them at this point, especially after the pandemic. It seems like flights get delayed more often, unless this is only my experience.

I'll also go food shopping and make sure I come home to a full fridge or freezer, if possible. If you're traveling for longer than a week, the fridge situation might not hold up, but you can put a few items in the freezer or cabinet for your return. You might be so exhausted that all you want to do is order takeout, and that's completely acceptable. Will takeout be there if your flight is delayed and you get in at three in the morning? Unlikely. Plan for the worst. I usually have a pizza in the freezer as a backup plan.

What's in the Bag

Okay, so what the hell do you pack for jet lag? Think about jet lag as something that will happen to you regardless, and you're packing stuff to make it suck less. You'll focus more on the stuff we talked about earlier, like sleeping arrangements and routines.

If I'm visiting family, I'll ask what they have for sleeping arrangements. If I'm going to be on a couch or in a place with less privacy, I'll bring a sleeping mask and earplugs. I'll use some pillows to create a barrier so it feels like my own space. I'll ask when people typically fall asleep because sometimes they may be in the living room longer than you'd expect even though you're exhausted and just want to fall asleep. If someone is used to sitting on the couch and watching TV, asking if there's another private place to chill before everyone falls asleep is helpful. If I can't find a place, I'll normally try to go for a walk outside if it's a safe part of town. You can unwind by walking and clearing your mind. Not ideal, of course, but better than sitting on the couch anxious about when people will go to sleep.

What's in my luggage? I'll pack my sleeping pillow for sure and a light blanket, if possible. I always bring a set of earplugs to ensure outside noise doesn't bother me. I'll download a white noise playlist to mimic the sounds of a fan that I usually have. I'll bring ice packs to pop in the freezer if I know I get a little hot at night. I bring a sleep mask, but if you don't have one, no stress. Just bring a dark-colored shirt to put over your eyes.

I'll also bring a pharmacy of drugs if I need it, such as ibuprofen, Benadryl, and Pepto Bismol, because you never know how you'll wake up after a night of traveling. I never expect people to have anything I need, so I pack it because I want to be prepared. Benadryl also acts as an OTC sleep aid, so it helps with allergic reactions or temporary sleep issues, which comes in handy when traveling.

I like to bring a reusable water bottle, too. You won't be able to get this on the plane if it's full, so empty it and throw it in your luggage. It's easier than grabbing cups in someone's house and wondering which cups are for who and if you're stepping on anybody's toes. I also bring snacks. A fuck ton of snacks that I like. These are relatively easy to pack because they don't take up too much space. You never know the eating schedule you'll be on; sometimes your friends and family only eat one or two meals a day and you might be used to eating three or four meals or snacking throughout the day.

Mimic Your Home Routine

The key is to try to mimic your home routine and situation as much as possible. It might not be perfect, but if you can get the sentiment of the activities you do at home, it's a win. If you usually wake up, brush your teeth, wash your face, and go for a light walk, try to do this when you're away. If it's not possible, maybe you can sit outside in the morning and get some fresh air, or stand in place while you make breakfast rather than sitting down. It's not the same, but it's similar enough. Try to do this every day if possible.

I keep my phone in my original time zone and have alarm clocks in the hotel room at the normal time to ensure I'm not late. I will usually set my watch to the current time zone, however. It gets tricky, so you'll have to figure out what works best for you. If it's ten o'clock in my original time zone and the current time is eight o'clock, I have no shame excusing myself to go to sleep if I'm exhausted. My goal is to stay in my original time zone to make it suck less when I get home.

When in Doubt: Hard Reset

If none of this is possible, you might want to do a hard reset when you return home. I try to get the earliest flight out so I have the entire day to decompress when I'm home. Since my house is workweek ready, I try to focus on prioritizing my sleep and reducing my stress. I might need to exist at home for a few hours and rejuvenate so that I'm ready for the workweek. I'm one of those people who empties their entire luggage and does the laundry on the same day. Does that make me weird? Probably. Does it help me regain a sense of stability after traveling? Absolutely.

You'll want to prioritize your sleep schedule once you're home. For acute and temporary jet lag, you might invest in some over-the-counter medications. You might get home and be wired because you were in the opposite time zone, so this may take a bit longer to get used to. The farther away you are from your original time zone, the more it might take to get back to normal. Be patient with your body.

I went to Australia to present research and my circadian rhythm was like, "What the actual hell is going on?" Australia is opposite from the United States in terms of seasons and time zones, so it was difficult to manage. I couldn't stay in my original time zone because it would have been the middle of the night when I ate breakfast. It was wild. So I focused most of my energy on readjusting when I returned. I remember lying in bed at night and being wide awake. Like, I could have run a few miles once my head hit the pillow—that's how awake I was. I invested in some OTC sleep aids to ease my body into readjusting, and it helped. I spoke with my doctor, and although it was a little weird at first, I only had to take it for a few days before my body was back to normal. Everyone's different, so you'll want to figure out what works for your situation.

Daylight Saving Time (DST)

Spring ahead and fall behind—cute, right? We've heard a lot about Daylight Saving Time and how we prepare for it every March and November. It's one of those uncontrollables that tends to wreck our sleep routine. When we gain an hour, I don't hear a lot of fuss. But when we lose an hour, it has the potential to wreck our sleep cycle. Even just an hour!

On top of that, there's research to suggest that DST reduces our sleep efficiency and duration.[221] There's also some knowledge that the clock shift in the spring is more detrimental to our sleep-wake cycle than when we shift the clocks in the fall, as researchers have noticed a reduction of time in bed (TIB) and total sleep time (TST), later wake times for our final awakening, and an increase in awakenings after we go to sleep (WASO).[222] This means that switching our clocks obviously messes with our circadian rhythm.

In insomnia treatment, I usually discuss with my clients how even one hour can potentially derail our sleep cycles. Our bodies are sensitive to even small changes. It's not to say we can't compensate for them, but it's important to keep this in mind as we navigate implementing healthy sleep habits.

"But what if this works the opposite way, and now I'm overly concerned about my sleep and losing even a few minutes?" We call that excessive sleep effort, which is sometimes a common natural consequence of sleep treatment. It's when we are overly rigid, anxious, and concerned about our sleep routine or sleep cycle. A for effort! But this might also cause some issues. Focusing too much time on our sleep is likely to cause anxiety, and we know that anxiety stops us from getting good sleep. It keeps us awake and makes it difficult to fall into a sleep routine. We lie awake for hours, wondering what we did wrong. The key is to focus on sleep but chill with it. It's like you're putting in the effort to make something change but you're not worried about the outcome.

---

221 Lahti, T. A., Leppämäki, S., Lönnqvist, J., and Partonen, T. (2006). Transition to daylight saving time reduces sleep duration plus sleep efficiency of the deprived sleep. *Neuroscience Letters, 406*(3), 174–177.

222 Tonetti, L., Erbacci, A., Fabbri, M., Martoni, M., and Natale, V. (2013). Effects of transitions into and out of daylight saving time on the quality of the sleep/wake cycle: An actigraphic study in healthy university students. *Chronobiology International, 30*(10), 1218–1222.

It's similar to going to college. You try to learn as much as you can in class without worrying about your test grades, like viewing grades as a natural consequence of learning. You use your grades to make changes, but you're not too concerned if you get an A or a B because both will suffice for passing the class. If you take a few small things from this class, you're likely to remember them and use that to navigate your career rather than trying to remember everything and making it perfect. We don't want it to be perfect. Perfect isn't real (in my opinion). We want it to be realistic and achievable, with a couple of fuckups along the way because it gives you character and edge. We'll talk more about this later when we chat about sleep expectations (my favorite part!).

Consequences of Permanent DST

The United States Senate approved a permanent daylight saving bill on March 15, 2022,[223] called the Sunshine Protection Act. This bill would eliminate our need to change the clocks to the standard time for the four months from November to March, so we wouldn't need to fall back on November 5, 2023.[224]

Tips if Your Location Still Observes DST

I specialize in sleep and didn't think it made much of a difference, but those four months of increased darkness affect me. I am less motivated to work or do things, and I barely want to leave the house because it's cold and dark. I want to eat more because I'm inside and I rarely go

223 Buckle, A., and Gunderson, M. (2022). *US Senate approves permanent DST bill*. TimeAndDate. https://www.timeanddate.com/news/time/us-permanent-dst.html.

224 117th Congress. (2022). *S.623- Sunshine Protection Act of 2021*. https://www.congress.gov/ bill/117th-congress/senate-bill/623/text.

to the gym in the winter because once it gets dark out, guess what? Those internal cues of sleepiness are *loud*. I'm sure most of you can relate to this.

So, what do we do until we don't have to switch our clocks again? Well, we have to roll with this somehow. I normally like to plan for DST switches and create a reminder in my calendar for the week before. If possible, I suggest prioritizing sleep health as the clocks push forward one hour. You'll miss an entire sixty minutes of sleep and still be required to function the next day. So, you'll either have to reduce your expectations for yourself the next day (e.g., not having as much energy, laying low, prioritizing relaxation after work if possible, etc.), or plan ahead of time to get to sleep a little earlier. The latter is usually difficult for people because they may not observe those internal cues of sleepiness earlier. If that's the case, you might have to allow yourself to be a little more tired the next day while prioritizing sleep the following night. Yes, this sounds effortful, but it's good for your health!

Chapter 5

ALCOHOL AND CANNABIS

I'm not trying to be a buzzkill here (no pun intended), but we have to talk about how alcohol and cannabis affect our sleep. As you know, I'm coming from a harm-reduction approach viewpoint, meaning I'm not going to tell you to simply stop using fun substances. There can be utility to these substances. I mean, hey, you're using them for a reason, right? It's a matter of how and when we're using them and if they're *actually* helpful. It's about being intentional with our choices because sometimes we realize we're doing things just, well, because we're doing them, not because they have inherent value.

Alcohol is everywhere, quite literally. It's in commercials. People talk about it. People ask you if you're drinking. People offer you drinks when you get to their homes. You might drink alone at night. You might struggle with alcohol addiction. If that's you, this book will touch on a few points that relate to sleep. However, alcohol addiction is serious, so contact your doctor before stopping completely because there can be fatal effects of giving it up cold turkey.

Cannabis has been the underdog for a while and has been becoming more mainstream as the years have gone on. A few people out there are cannabis haters, and if you're one of them, you might as well just skip this chapter. Well, I mean, stick around if you feel comfortable. You might learn some good stuff!

My hope is that we can take a deeper look into how these substances affect our sleep to make some helpful life changes. It might mean cutting back a little, choosing different drinks, or consuming them at different times. It's sometimes hard to imagine life without substances because we rely on them for certain things. Maybe you use them to feel less anxious in social situations or you believe they help you sleep at night. This makes sense but you're not letting your body feel the anxiety so you can work through it.

Taking the edge off is helpful at times, though. It's like therapy. We talk about trauma and sometimes we use humor to get through it. Is humor helpful as the only way to get through things? Maybe. Is it helpful to dig deep into trauma? Sometimes. It might hold you back, but it's helpful in small amounts. That's how I see substances, so if this checks out for you, keep reading.

Alcohol

We touched on alcohol briefly when we discussed nightly awakenings, and I think it's worth exploring more in this chapter. You've probably heard people say, "A few drinks help me fall asleep." Part of this is true. We know that alcohol is a central nervous system (CNS) depressant, meaning it slows our brain activity.[225] The CNS, which is composed of the brain and spinal cord, is responsible for sending and receiving messages between the body and brain. Alcohol affects these messages by slowing them down, thus affecting our attention, concentration, processing speed, and coordination.

Depending on the dosage, people who drink large amounts of alcohol might notice slurred speech, trouble walking, and changes in

---

225 Vezali Costardi, J. V., Teruaki Nampo, R. A., Silva, G. L., Ferreira Ribeiro, M. A., Stella, H. J., Stella, M. B., and Pinheiro Malheiros, S. V. (2015). A review on alcohol: From the central action mechanism to chemical dependency. *Revista da Associação Médica Brasileira, 61,* 381-387.

breathing and mood. They may not process information like they do when they're sober. Have you ever had a little too much to drink and reacted negatively to a situation? Then you wake up the next morning like, "Why was I even upset about that?" or "Wow, I hope I didn't say anything stupid."

Of course, there are reasons why people drink alcohol. They believe it helps them become more relaxed; they might not feel physical or emotional pain quite like they do when they're sober. Alcohol also might reduce anxiety in certain social situations (a.k.a. "liquid courage"). And I wish they didn't, but some people also use alcohol to help with their sleep. Although alcohol may cause sleepiness, it has the potential to wreck our sleep quality and total sleep duration.[226] Researchers suggest that alcohol may suppress REM sleep during the earlier parts of the sleep cycle, resulting in a REM rebound effect. Okay, so what the hell does this mean?

Remember when we talked about sleep cycles and different stages of sleep? (See page 74.) There's REM and then non-REM stages 1, 2, and 3. For the first few cycles at the beginning of the night, we notice we usually spend more time in deeper stages of sleep, then we notice we get more REM sleep as the night progresses because our bodies are preparing for final awakening. We still need REM sleep in the beginning, just not as much. Well, alcohol suppresses this REM sleep at the beginning of the night, resulting in an imbalance of deep sleep and REM sleep. This means that our sleep architecture is jacked up, and we wake up feeling unrested and may have more awakenings overnight. You might also notice that you wake up feeling generally unrested and hungover, so you'll likely take a nap. And boy, that nap is

226 Park, S., Oh, M., Lee, B., Kim, H., Lee, W., Lee, J., Lim, J., and Kim, J. (2015). The effects of alcohol on quality of sleep. *Korean Journal of Family Medicine, 36*(6), 294-299.

refreshing! That's probably because your body is trying to catch up on
that lack of REM.

Those who drink alcohol in excess (a.k.a. binge drinking) may have
issues falling and staying asleep. There's a link between alcohol and
sleep difficulties, and I tend to wonder if alcohol does more than mess
up our sleep cycle and architecture. Have you ever drunk and then
woke up sweating overnight? What about feeling flushed in the face
when you drink? I had a feeling alcohol affected thermoregulation
(a.k.a. our ability to regulate our core temperature), so I did
some digging.

Alcohol is a vasodilator, meaning it widens our blood vessels, resulting
in more blood flow to our skin.[227] This makes us feel flushed and hot,
which increases our skin temperature. As a result, we start sweating
because that helps our body cool down. Well, this might affect you as
you sleep because if you feel hot and flushed, you might wake up more
often. Remember we talked about how your core body temperature
drops a little overnight while you sleep? Well, a once natural process
is now a tug-of-war because alcohol is pumping through your
bloodstream. You might also wake up more to use the bathroom
because alcohol is a toxin, and your body is flushing it out and trying
to survive. Your body's top priority is getting rid of the toxin (alcohol)
rather than focusing on all the other stuff it has to do while it sleeps
(cue in our earlier chapter about what our body does as it sleeps).
Yes, let's focus on this for a minute—alcohol is a literal toxin. It has
no benefit for our body. We *think* it's helping us sleep or calming us
down, but really, our body is desperately trying to rid itself of alcohol
because it's harmful to us.

---

227 Davis, A., and Jarvis, S. (202). *How does alcohol affect your body temperature?* Patient. https://
patient.info/news-and-features/how-does-alcohol-affect-your-body-temperature.

Another thing to consider is that alcohol changes your brain chemistry. Go into Google Images and type in "differences between non-drinker and binge drinker brain." You're welcome for some nightmares. The image I'm thinking of comes from Cierra Foley, guest writer for *The Egalitarian*.[228] If alcohol changes the functionality of our brain, I can't even imagine what we don't know about how it affects sleep. Sheeeesh!

Basically, you drink some alcohol, your body says, "Oh shit, here's an intruder," and it orchestrates this event to get the toxin out. You're hanging out on your couch, and you start to feel the sedative effects, meanwhile, your body is freaking out internally, trying to maintain everything. "Everybody, stay calm!" So you think it's going to help you with your sleep, but your body desperately needs to get rid of it.

What is the cost of doing this every night? You don't get into the stages of sleep that you need to at the right times, you wake up more, you feel flushed, and you don't sleep as long or as deeply. What's the point? Some people have anxiety about sleep, and they believe alcohol helps them feel a sense of calmness. But those few drinks might cost you quality sleep. In my opinion, I'd rather experience anxiety before bed and have trouble falling asleep, but when I do sleep, at least I know my body won't have to work extra hard. You might notice that you don't sleep as long when you don't drink alcohol. Well, that may be true, and your body may have to do less work in fewer hours because it doesn't have to worry about a toxin. All this, and you don't have to worry about a hangover.

One thing I will say is that alcohol isn't a substance that you can abstain from if you've been drinking a lot. In fact, if you are a heavy

---

228 Foley, C. *Speaker raises awareness on alcohol abuse*. The Egalitarian. https://hccegalitarian.com/2403/showcase/speaker-raises-awareness-on-alcohol-abuse/?print=true.

drinker or someone who drinks every day, you'll seriously want to consider chatting with your doctor before reducing your alcohol intake. Yeah, you might have some unpleasant withdrawal effects, but some people risk their lives by abstaining.[229] Extremely heavy drinkers who stop drinking randomly may experience seizures or delirium tremens (DT), which can be fatal. Yeah, fatal as in you can die. Big yikes. Even worse, if someone is withdrawing from alcohol and they fall asleep, they are unaware of their symptoms and this can happen overnight. You see where I'm going with this.

This indirectly relates to our sleep. One of the symptoms of alcohol withdrawal is anxiety. Anxiety is one of those factors we talked about earlier that inhibit us from falling asleep soundly. If we're anxious about something, we're less likely to fall asleep quickly. Another withdrawal symptom of quitting alcohol if you're a heavy drinker is insomnia. When people stop drinking completely, they may have issues sleeping, which is why I think some people don't want to quit in the first place. This goes away over time. A physical symptom that may affect sleep is headaches or migraines. Of course, we can take over-the-counter medication for this, but it's still unpleasant and causes issues with falling asleep, too.

My overall take on alcohol: the negative effects might outweigh the benefits, but everything in moderation. Drinking one drink every now and then might not be terrible for your health, but drinking every night to go to sleep might not be the best idea. If people do want to drink, I often suggest trying to avoid alcohol before bedtime. If you're the type to meet your friends for drinks, going for happy hour or lunch on the weekend might be a safe bet. When we drink right before bed, it might affect our sleep cycles.

---

229 Watkins, M. (2022). *Risks & dangers of quitting alcohol cold turkey.* American Addiction Centers. https://americanaddictioncenters.org/withdrawal-timelines-treatments/cold-turkey.

Marijuana (Cannabis)

Good ol' marijuana. Cannabis. Weed. Pot. Whatever we call it nowadays, it's gained traction in the media and medical field. There are states legalizing medical and recreational cannabis, and some countries are exploring how cannabis can help with medical conditions. But can it help with sleep?

Before you continue reading this, let me clear the air. This isn't going to be a chapter that's black-and-white when it comes to cannabis. I'm going to talk about the research and let you make your decision, as this can be a charged topic for some people. I'm not a medication prescriber and certainly not a budtender (a.k.a. people who work at medical marijuana dispensaries). Therefore, I am not a cannabis expert, but as with any new development, I am interested to see if it works for sleep as a harm-reduction approach. Psychologists are interested in being up-to-date with the research, and if this can be helpful, we lean into these research studies to learn more.

This will go without saying, but anything that we chat about here is for your information to bring to your doctor or healthcare specialist. I suggest speaking with your doctor before making any decisions about your health, especially when it comes to cannabis because everyone's healthcare issues are unique and there's no one-size-fits-all. I'm here to relay the research because it's something my clients and friends ask me about all the time. This is a book about sleep, not a book about cannabis, but it's important to see if there's a connection here. Therefore, the level of detail won't be the same if you're reading a book about cannabis. So, we will discuss a few key points for educational purposes, then get to the research, which is still developing as we speak.

Why Cannabis and Sleep?

The questions about cannabis have become unavoidable, and not going to lie, I was apprehensive about diving deep into this subject because I didn't know much about it until a few years ago. I've seen it work wonders for some people, but not everyone. So, I did a ton of research and talked to as many people as I could about how it helped or didn't help them. The research varies depending on the country, laws, and politics. There's still a lot we don't know, but I'm going to share what I've discovered as it relates to sleep. This research interest didn't happen out of nowhere—something sparked this.

There was a *huge* turning point for me in how I viewed weed, and it was kind of unexpected. No, I didn't have a crazy trip or anything. One of my best friends was in the army and she sustained a traumatic brain injury (TBI) while deployed in Iraq. She started having seizures out of nowhere. She wasn't the same when she came back, even though she appeared somewhat normal (honestly, what even is normal nowadays, though?). She's pretty, physically fit, and generally appears able and functioning. But she struggled.

It's demoralizing to watch your friend go through something so difficult. The complications of her TBI seem to be the cause of her epileptic seizures. She never had a seizure before this deployment. She had a rough upbringing, but who doesn't have childhood trauma? After a decade of testing, medication trials, and therapy, she approached me and was like, "I just can't take it anymore. Nothing's working, not even the medications." I saw my best friend go from feeling empowered to feeling completely shattered by this condition. Then, she got her medical marijuana card. I can't even tell you the last time she had a seizure because it's been that long. She's also sleeping way better. Her sleep is honestly pristine. Her body has those internal cues of sleepiness, and her circadian rhythm is predictable; she wakes up at the same time every day. She's experimented with medications again here and there, but she always goes back to the one thing that never failed her when all the other doctors did: cannabis.

I was like, "Holy fuck, this shit actually works." That started my journey of researching more and more about cannabis, THC, CBD, and cannabinoids in general. I kept thinking, *How does this relate to sleep?* It has to impact sleep somehow. I know that OTC medications and some prescription medications can make insomnia worse or cause serious side effects. Does cannabis do that, too? What if cannabis can assist with sleep but reduce the side effects if someone is interested in using medication or substances for sleep?

Most of us have experimented with *something*. Whether it's legal is another story. Maybe it's weed, alcohol, illicit substances, or hallucinogens. Maybe it's acid or ecstasy. Maybe it's caffeine. Maybe it's not even a substance, but it's something out of the ordinary, like doing a 5k on a holiday. Kidding, I'm definitely not one of those overachievers on holidays. If you are, how do you get motivated to do this? That might be a question for another day.

Anyway, substances exist to enhance high or low moments; maybe they cause destruction. Maybe they cause euphoria, help us get through certain moments in life, or foster connection or a sense of purpose. Maybe they foster addiction and disconnection from our loved ones. Regardless, it's important to talk about marijuana because it has been around for a while, and it might affect sleep.

For the purposes of this book, I'm mostly going to talk about medical marijuana, the kind that you get at a medical dispensary. These dispensaries can only provide marijuana to patients who have a medical marijuana card. They have access to marijuana due to certain conditions, and it requires a doctor's approval. You know I love data and research, and sometimes when we talk about recreational marijuana from an unknown source (e.g., insert your weed/drug dealer's name here), we don't exactly know the dosage, what else it's laced with, and if it's what the dealer says it is.

I'm sure your weed dealer is a great person, but they are not a double-blind, randomized, controlled trial that explores multiple facets of how this interacts with medical conditions and sleep. For those who aren't familiar with what a double-blind study is, you'll want to know why it's important. A double-blind study is when the researcher and the participant do not know if the participant is in the control group or the experimental group.[230] The experimental group is usually the group receiving the intervention (in this case, it would be a substance). The control group usually receives a placebo. This helps reduce bias within the study. It's almost like nobody knows what's going on, but the study was created and structured in a way that this information is revealed at the end of the trial.

Down to the Basics

A brief lesson on the mechanics and origins of marijuana is important because it's one of the most widely used recreational drugs. There are plenty of people still locked up for marijuana charges, which ignites a rage response in my soul because recreational marijuana is becoming legal in more states as the years go on. Yet, these people are still sitting in prison for something that's readily accessible to laypeople. I know it's not this simple, but it still baffles me.

---

230 National Cancer Institute. *Double-blind study*. NCI Dictionaries. https://www.cancer.gov/publications/dictionaries/cancer-terms/def/double-blind-study.

So, there are lot of politics and biases out there, but what the hell is marijuana? I recently learned that cannabis and marijuana aren't exactly the same thing. Cannabis comes from the plant Cannabis Sativa, and marijuana refers to the psychoactive parts of Cannabis Sativa, also known as tetrahydrocannabinol (THC).[231] THC is responsible for making you high; if you've ever taken it, you know that feeling. Some cannabis plants contain a lot of THC, and some don't contain so much. The ones with traces of THC (usually less than 0.3 percent of THC or less)[232] that aren't as pronounced are characterized as industrial hemp.

No, no, no. I'm not suggesting getting blitzed to get to sleep every night. It's simply helpful to understand the relationship between cannabis and sleep.

Our Endocannabinoid System

What is the endocannabinoid system? It's in our bodies. Ooo, kinda freaky, right? But our body has cannabinoid receptors (CB1 and CB2), and some sources say there are more of these receptors than any other receptor types in our brains.[233] Our bodies produce endocannabinoids, which are molecules extremely similar to the molecules in a cannabis plant. For an analogy, you know how we talked about how our body produces melatonin? Well, we can take exogenous melatonin that appears to be a similar structure, even though it's already created in our body. It's similar to this, only it's cannabis.

---

231 National Center for Complementary and Integrative Health. (2019). *Cannabis (marijuana) and cannabinoids: What you need to know.* U.S. Department of Health and Human Services. https://www.nccih.nih.gov/health/cannabis-marijuana-and-cannabinoids-what-you-need-to-know.

232 Holland, K. (2022). *CBD vs. THC: What's the difference?* Healthline. https://www.healthline.com/health/cbd-vs-thc.

233 Grinspoon, P. (2021). *The endocannabinoid system: Essential and mysterious.* Harvard Health Publishing. https://www.health.harvard.edu/blog/the-endocannabinoid-system-essential-and-mysterious-202108112569.

What do these cannabinoid receptors do? Well, they're basically like helicopter moms. They control the activity of other molecules, and they want to know everything about what the other receptors are doing. They help with a bunch of stuff, including regulating the activity of other molecules' systems for hunger, temperature, and other bodily functions. They're kind of a big deal, which is why I wanted to touch on them before we got talking about cannabinoids like CBD and THC.

CBD and THC

Again, not exactly a cannabis expert here, but I'll tell you what I know. Cannabis plants contain cannabinoids, which are broken up into two main parts: THC and Cannabidiol (CBD). There are hundreds of different types of cannabinoids; it honestly makes my head spin. THC and CBD are most cited in the research, so let's focus on these two for simplicity. THC and CBD both contain twenty-one carbon atoms, thirty hydrogen atoms, and two oxygen atoms, and the arrangement of these atoms is the reason why they both feel different when you take them (a.k.a. THC has more psychoactive effects compared to CBD).

Okay, story time. So CBD and THC enter your body. Almost immediately, they need to find their friends (kinda like you when you show up at a party and see a bunch of unfamiliar faces). The friends they're searching for are your cannabinoid receptors. Once they find the cannabinoid crew, they give them a big hug, but THC seems to stay attached. THC is a friend that gives too long of a hug; it's awkward but well-received. THC binds with the cannabinoid 1 (CB1) receptor in the brain, which is the reason we feel high. CBD isn't a love-bomber, so it sort of gives a handshake to CB1 to reduce some of the unwanted psychoactive effects produced by THC. CBD is the friend that shows up at the party, mostly as a supporter of THC. You notice their presence, but they're not in your face.

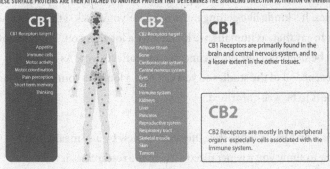

Human Endocannabinoid System

THE MOST WELL KNOWN CANNABINOID RECEPTORS, CB1 AND CB2, ARE PROTEINS THAT ARE IMBEDDED IN THE MEMBRANE OF CELLS.
THESE SURFACE PROTEINS ARE THEN ATTACHED TO ANOTHER PROTEIN THAT DETERMINES THE SIGNALING DIRECTION ACTIVATION OR INHIBITION

CB1
CB1 Receptors target :
Appetite
Immune cells
Motor activity
Motor coordination
Pain perception
Short term memory
Thinking

CB2
CB2 Receptors target :
Adipose tissue
Bone
Cardiovascular system
Central nervous system
Eyes
Gut
Immune system
Kidneys
Liver
Pancreas
Reproductive system
Respiratory tract
Skeletal muscle
Skin
Tumors

CB1
CB1 Receptors are primarily found in the brain and central nervous system, and to a lesser extent in the other tissues.

CB2
CB2 Receptors are mostly in the peripheral organs especially cells associated with the immune system.

This process affects the neurotransmitters in our brain, which are responsible for sending and receiving messages from certain cells that affect certain roles in our body, including pain, sleep, or stress. There are also different strains, including Sativa, Indica, and hybrids (usually a mixture of Sativa and Indica). People can take cannabis in the form of oils, edibles, tinctures, capsules, and smoke it from a vape or flower.[234] The mode of administration depends on your comfort, how long you want it to last, and what you're using it for. Now that you understand the chemical reaction behind these substances, let's dive into what the research says about them.

---

234 See footnote 233.

The Research

I like looking at substances as they relate to the presenting issue (sleep) and comorbid conditions (e.g., anxiety, depression). Sometimes we experience both depression and insomnia, and sometimes it's only insomnia. Either way, it's helpful to see if a substance will help reduce symptomology for the specific issue or if it will help with a host of issues. It's kinda like getting more bang for your buck. I think it's also fair to say that, as humans, we kinda have a lot going on. It might not just be sleep, but our other concerns may affect sleep. As always, I'll reference all of the studies so you can take a look for yourself. The key here is to be well-informed.

This won't be an exhaustive literature review by any means, but I want to show you a generalized view of the research as it relates to marijuana and mental health, substance use, and sleep because they're all connected. Like I've said before, it's important to consider that a lot of these research studies are relatively new, have limited sample sizes, may be subject to bias, and are sometimes limited depending on the funding and location. We can still derive some good data points from these studies because scientists and researchers work hard at making this information readily available to us. It's kind of their job. As for me, I'm pretty neutral on the topic so I'm going to provide a viewpoint that may not be on one side or the other. For me, it usually depends on the person's goals and what they're using medical marijuana for.

An important consideration is that many studies may not be able to identify direct causation. Meaning it might not be able to directly link cannabis to a reduction or exacerbation of mental health symptoms, just like we're not sure that eating terribly directly causes heart attacks. We know that our diet and lifestyle habits certainly affect our overall health outlook, and this may create a higher likelihood of cardiovascular issues. However, we are never certain. There's not usually one single cause. Same goes for cannabis research. It might be helpful to see that cannabis reduces symptom severity, duration, or frequency, but sometimes it's truly hard to tell if it's cannabis or something else.

Another consideration is that we currently have limited studies on cannabis and there may be inherent biases within the research itself. For example, medical cannabis isn't federally regulated, and people have mixed feelings about cannabis in general. Some people are big supporters because it helps from a harm-reduction approach. This means that cannabis may help more than harm, and it helps people regain their lives without using prescription medications with big side effects.

Other people still see cannabis as a drug that may be abused. Of course, there are always ways that anything can be abused. I tend to view this from an individualized perspective. It's not for everyone, and everyone may need different things. If it works for you and it's not causing harm, great! If you've talked to your medical doctor about it and you've seen that it can help alleviate certain symptoms, even better. However, if your doctor advises against it, it might be for a good reason. Regardless, there's no one-size-fits-all with marijuana, so seeing the research this way is important.

Marijuana and Mental Health

Ah, so this comes up a lot in therapy. I'll meet with someone for an intake and ask about substance use, and they'll hesitate because they don't know how I feel about it. If you're going to use it, you may as well be informed, so let's figure out how you can do so in a safe and effective way. We've seen that asking people to abstain from these substances doesn't work so well because they may feel shame or think they're being judged. Worst-case scenario, they leave therapy and never come back. That doesn't help anyone, does it?

We know that mental health, substance use, and sleep are interconnected. When we are experiencing anxiety, depression, or triggers from past trauma, it might impact our sleep. Have you ever laid in bed and couldn't get to sleep because you keep remembering that thing that's happened to you? You wish it never happened. Or maybe you're trying to think about how to grow through it. I often have these moments when my head hits the pillow, and I'm sure you can relate. And no, I'm not saying to get high as hell off marijuana and float into your bed and go to Mars instead of going to sleep. If you do, I won't judge you. I'm here to say that we try to do a lot to manage our mental health when we're struggling, and medical marijuana might be something to consider to take the edge off.

PTSD

We noticed from the research that THC and CBD have been used to help those with nightmares resulting from post-traumatic stress disorder (PTSD),[235] and some people didn't meet the criteria for a PTSD diagnosis after a while.[236] Importantly, THC and CBD may help reduce hyperarousal, which, as mentioned earlier, can impact sleep quality. Isn't this wild?

---

235 Kaul, M., Zee, P.C. and Sahni, A.S. (2021). Effects of cannabinoids on sleep and their therapeutic potential for sleep disorders. *Neurotherapeutics, 18,* 217-227.

236 Bonn-Miller, M. O., Brunstetter, M., Simonian, A., Loflin, M. J., Vandrey, R., Babson, K. A., and Wortzel, H. (2022). The long-term, prospective, therapeutic impact of cannabis on post-traumatic stress disorder. *Cannabis and Cannabinoid Research, 7*(2), 214-223.

Anxiety and Depression

Let's look at anxiety, depression, and marijuana through the lens of a meta-analysis, which is a systematic review of multiple studies. The one that I'm thinking of in particular analyzed data from thirteen studies that included six thousand participants from thirty countries who were using medical cannabis for pain, depression, or anxiety.[237] Damn, that's a lot of people smoking weed. Researchers found that there was substantial evidence to support the use of cannabis for those experiencing pain but mixed results for anxiety. People may experience relief from anxiety symptoms, but they may increase after people stop using cannabis completely. As for depression, cannabis was shown to be helpful in reducing symptoms, and this was true for people even after a one-year follow-up.

Substance Use

What about other substances that affect mental health and sleep? Well, since the inception of medical marijuana, we've seen opioid deaths decrease dramatically in the United States.[238] A survey in 2017 explored substance use and medical marijuana use among dispensary patients, and it showed a significant reduction in opioid use. In fact, 75 percent of the patients who regularly used opioids used medical cannabis instead.[239] Interestingly, 42 percent of those who used alcohol reduced their use or used medical marijuana instead. The accessibility of medical marijuana may reduce overdoses, DUI deaths, and other physical health complications with extended use of opioids or alcohol.

---

237 Danielsson, A., Lundin, A., Agardh, E., Allebeck, P., and Forsell, Y. (2016). Cannabis use, depression and anxiety: A 3-year prospective population-based study. *Journal of Affective Disorders, 193*, 103–108.

238 Piper, B. J., DeKeuster, R. M., Beals, M. L, Cobb, C. M., Burchman, C. A., Perkinson, L., Lynn, S. T., Nichols, S. D., and Abess, A. T. (2017). Substitution of medical cannabis for pharmaceutical agents for pain, anxiety and sleep. *Journal of Psychopharmacology, 31*(5), 569–575.

239 See footnote 239.

Marijuana and Sleep

Does it help or does it not help with sleep? Well, it depends. Research on marijuana and sleep is still in its infancy, which means we have a long way to go. It's important to note some of the limitations here. Many clinical studies from the past have relatively small sample sizes (meaning there are not many participants included in the study, which makes it hard to generalize to the greater population). However, these studies have suggested there may be a therapeutic benefit to cannabinoids for managing certain sleep issues. There are studies for insomnia and OSA (Obstructive Sleep Apnea), but there needs to be more clinical research at larger levels. It would be helpful to include dosing, efficacy levels, and safety considerations for certain types of cannabinoids as they relate to sleep.

Remember we talked briefly about CB1 before, the receptor that THC was obsessed with? Well, CB1 helps with launching the sleep process.[240] Basically, serotonergic neurons (a.k.a. serotonin, that neurotransmitter we all love) help with regulating sleep-wake cycles.[241] There are studies that show endocannabinoids modulate our serotonin system and CB1 receptors help regulate that process.[242, 243] Like we discussed earlier, CBD and THC have different relationships with CB1 and CB2, suggesting that there are different psychoactive effects, which may also impact our sleep.[244] Okay, so how does this affect sleep specifically?

---

240 Murillo-Rodríguez, E. (2008). The role of the CB1 receptor in the regulation of sleep. *Progress in Neuro-Psychopharmacology and Biological Psychiatry, 32*(6),1420–1427.

241 Maejima, T., Masseck, O. A., Mark, M. D., and Herlitze, S. (2013). Modulation of firing and synaptic transmission of serotonergic neurons by intrinsic G protein-coupled receptors and ion channels. *Frontiers in Integrative Neuroscience, 7*, 40.

242 Devlin, M. G., and Christopoulos, A. (2002). Modulation of cannabinoid agonist binding by 5-HT in the rat cerebellum. *Journal of Neurochemistry, 80*(6),1095–1102.

243 Fan, P. (1995). Cannabinoid agonists inhibit the activation of 5-HT3 receptors in rat nodose ganglion neurons. *Journal of Neurophysiology, 73*(2), 907–910.

244 See footnote 236.

Let's talk about different frequencies and dosing as they relate to our sleep architecture. A research review from Kaul, Zee, and Sahni (2021) outlines these effects perfectly, as they detail the effects of THC and cannabis and provide a summary of the research. So, this isn't just their study, but they considered other research studies, too. As always, this is referenced if you'd like to do your own reading, which I highly recommend. These researchers also provide visuals about how THC affects our sleep hypnogram (a map of our sleep architecture and what stages of sleep we're in and how THC may impact this).[245]

THC

From an acute standpoint, meaning only using a substance for a short period of time, we notice that people seem to obtain more consolidated sleep when they use THC. This means they have fewer awakenings overnight and more consecutive hours of sleep. It reduces sleep latency, a.k.a. the time it takes us to fall asleep when our head hits the pillow. We notice less REM sleep and more deep sleep. But here's the kicker: they aren't using THC every single night for weeks or years.

From a chronic use standpoint, meaning using THC for an extended period, the effects may be different. It's honestly kind of shocking to think that acute and long-term use changes the way that THC affects our sleep and our bodies. We notice that there is less deep sleep, more frequent awakenings, it may take a bit longer to fall asleep, and it reduces our total sleep time. Holy shit, what? Remember the saying, "Only do things in moderation"? I think this is what they mean.

---

245 See footnote 236.

CBD

There's a limited amount of studies that show the effect of CBD on sleep in humans; however, researchers reported that CBD might increase total sleep time in rats.[246, 247] A more recent study showed increased internal cues of sleepiness upon CBD administration, but researchers were unsure how much THC was involved, so it's hard to say if it was solely the effect of CBD.[248] So, we might need more study in this area to say if CBD helps with sleep for sure.

Sleep-Wake Cycle

We've seen how THC and CBD may affect our sleep overnight, but how does it affect our overall sleep-wake cycle, a.k.a. our circadian rhythm? We know that consistency with our routines and exposure to light may affect wakefulness or sleepiness, and cannabinoids may have a role here. We chatted about this earlier, but if we're talking about marijuana, it warrants a quick review. Our hypothalamus contains a structure called the suprachiasmatic nucleus (SCN), which regulates our sleep-wake cycle. Well, guess what? The CB1 receptor (the receptor that THC is obsessed with) may affect this cycle, and we know that CB1 has a role in the endocannabinoid system.[249] We're seeing some connections here.

---

246 Chagas, M. H. N., Crippa, J. A. S., Zuardi, A. W., Hallak, J. E. C., Machado-de-Sousa, J. M., Hirotsu, C., Maia, L., Tufik, S., and Andersen, M. L. (2013). Effects of acute systemic administration of cannabidiol on sleep-wake cycle in rats. *Journal of Psychopharmacology, 27*(3), 312–316.

247 Monti, J. M. (1977). Hypnoticlike effects of cannabidiol in the rat. *Psychopharmacology, 55*(3), 263–265.

248 Spindle, T. R., Cone, E. J., Goffi, E., Weerts, E. M., Mitchell, J. M., Winecker, R. E., Bigelow, G. E., Flegel, R. R., and Vandrey, R. (2020). Pharmacodynamic effects of vaporized and oral cannabidiol (CBD) and vaporized CBD-dominant cannabis in infrequent cannabis users. *Drug Alcohol Dependence, 211,* 107937.

249 See footnote 236.

Animals may have lower levels of endocannabinoids when exposed to bright lights (they feel awake) and increased amounts when it's dark (they are sleepy). It shows us that this endocannabinoid system is related to animals' circadian rhythm. It's not only melatonin and other stuff, but these endocannabinoids may also affect the sleep-wake cycle in rodents.[250, 251] But what about us?

Research has shown that THC alone may not have a huge effect on our circadian rhythms related to falling asleep and may be more responsible for disrupting sleep architecture (a.k.a. how long we are in certain stages of sleep and how often these sleep stages occur).[252] In other words, it affects our sleep quality in some ways. But some researchers found that THC may help reduce apneas overnight (a.k.a. periods of non-breathing).[253, 254] This also depends on if we're considering THC for short- or long-term use because, as we've discussed, the side effects are pretty drastic.

Indirect Effects on Our Sleep Cycle

Relatedly, I know you've heard about people getting the munchies after taking THC. This may also affect our circadian rhythm. Our endocannabinoid system is also involved in regulating our appetite, particularly the reward system involved in eating, even when we don't

250 Sanford, A. E., Castillo, E., and Gannon, R. L. (2008). Cannabinoids and hamster circadian activity rhythms. *Brain Research, 1222,* 141-148.

251 Acuna-Goycolea, C., Obrietan, K., and van den Pol, A. N. (2010). Cannabinoids excite circadian clock neurons. *Journal of Neuroscience, 30*(30), 10061-10066.

252 Monti, J. M., and Pandi-Perumal, S. R. (2022). Clinical management of sleep and sleep disorders with cannabis and cannabinoids: Implications to practicing psychiatrists. *Clinical Neuropharmacology, 45*(2), 27-31.

253 Farabi, S. S., Prasad, B., Quinn, L., and Carley, D. W. (2014). Impact of dronabinol on quantitative electroencephalogram (qEEG) measures of sleep in obstructive sleep apnea syndrome. *Journal of Clinical Sleep Medicine, 10*(1), 49-56.

254 See footnote 253.

have internal cues of hunger.[255] So if we're taking THC, it's likely to disrupt that. Not because THC is to blame, but because of the side effects, such as how much we're eating. We know that when we eat at certain times of the day, it has the potential to disrupt our sleep, which isn't a direct effect of THC but an indirect side effect of using this substance.

Then, there's sleep debt. Good ol' sleep debt. It's that fancy term for the sleep we wish we obtained. Basically, sleep debt is the amount of sleep that we lose out on versus the amount of sleep we actually get. So if you're used to sleeping seven hours per night, but you only sleep five hours Monday through Friday, then you have a sleep debt of ten hours by Saturday morning. Yikes!

Some researchers suggest that we're more likely to eat energy-dense foods when we encounter sleep debt, which may be regulated by the endocannabinoid system. So, if our sleep is jacked up and we're not getting enough of it, we're likely to eat denser (and potentially unhealthier) foods because our endocannabinoid system highlights the need for more excessive food intake during this time.[256]

Medical Marijuana and Insomnia

Tons of research is still in progress right now. Researchers and scientists are working hard to pump out data on sleep, THC, and CBD, especially in the United States. So while we know what we know for now, there's still a lot out there that's a big question mark. My primary question is, does THC or CBD have any therapeutic effect on sleep

255 Coccurello, R., and Maccarrone M. (2018). Hedonic eating and the "delicious circle": From lipid-derived mediators to brain dopamine and Back. *Frontiers in Neuroscience, 12*, 271.

256 Hanlon, E. C., Tasali, E., Leproult, R., Stuhr, K. L., Doncheck, E., de Wit, H., Hillard, C. J., and Van Cauter, E. Sleep restriction enhances the daily rhythm of circulating levels of endocannabinoid 2-arachidonoylglycerol. (2016). *Sleep, 39*(3), 653–64.

disorders? These are disorders that have already been diagnosed by a professional. Let's find out.

Let's focus on the big fish and my favorite sleep disorder, insomnia. We know the first-line treatment for chronic insomnia is CBT-I, a combination of cognitive and behavioral treatments designed to help people make lasting lifestyle changes and sleep hygiene changes. Your insomnia is chronic, and these therapy modalities are iconic. Okay, *cringe*, moving on. We know that certain prescription and over-the-counter medications aren't always helpful for long-lasting insomnia. What about cannabinoids?

Cannabinoids tend to have a calming effect,[257] which means they may reduce anxiety. We know that anxiety, worry, and physiological arousal may keep us up and inhibit us from falling asleep quickly or soundly. We've known this for a while, as this has been cited in works dating as far back as the 1800s.[258, 259, 260] In 2017, a survey showed that 65 percent of 1,500 medical marijuana patients in a New England clinic reduced their prescription sleep medication due to using medical cannabis.[261]

However, reports suggest withdrawing from chronic use of marijuana may cause a rebound insomnia effect. Sounds scary. Well, it's not pleasant. One study found that withdrawing from marijuana may pose difficulty for sleep maintenance and initiation, meaning it may cause more issues falling and staying asleep once the person abstains from

---

257 Kesner, A. J., and Lovinger, D. M. (2020). Cannabinoids, endocannabinoids and sleep. *Frontiers in Molecular Neuroscience, 13*, 125.

258 Clendinning, J. (1843). Observations on the medicinal properties of the Cannabis Sativa of India. *Medico-Chirurgical Transactions, 26*, 188-210.

259 O'Shaughnessy, W. B. (1843). On the preparations of the Indian hemp, or Gunjah. *Provincial Medical Journal and the Retrospect of Medical Sciences, 5*(123), 363-369.

260 Wallich, G. C. (1883). Cannabis indica. *The British Medical Journal, 1*, 1224.

261 See footnote 239.

using marijuana.[262] So, we can gather that chronic use of marijuana may not be helpful for sleep, especially if we stop using it. Our body needs time to get used to the lack of substance, and it may suck for a little while.

Another study suggested that although the research between marijuana and sleep is relatively new, marijuana may help with insomnia, depending on the dose.[263] Researchers wanted to see the differences between daily and non-daily marijuana users. Half of the participants were white and were, on average, twenty-two years old. They used a few questionnaires for sleep that I use in my practice, like the Insomnia Severity Index Score (one of the big ones), Pittsburgh Sleep Quality Index, Epworth Sleepiness Scale, and the Morningness-Eveningness Questionnaire. These tools assess subjective sleep measures, meaning they are self-report questionnaires. Objective measures would include a polysomnography (a.k.a. data that isn't self-reported but can be gathered from a machine of some sort). Anyway, for non-daily users (a.k.a. people who did not use marijuana every day), their insomnia scores were lower than those who used marijuana daily. This means that those who didn't use marijuana every day seemed to have less issues falling or staying asleep.[264]

What about CBT-I and marijuana combined? A study in *The Journal of Clinical Sleep Medicine* found that regardless of cannabis use, those who engaged in CBT-I would find relief for insomnia symptoms. This means that those who use cannabis can still achieve helpful benefits from going through a CBT-I program to assist with sleep, even if they're drinking alcohol during this time. In fact, researchers identified

---

262 Kolla, B. P., Hayes, L., Cox,C., Eatwell, L., Deyo-Svendsen, M., and Mansukhani, M. P. (2022). The effects of cannabinoids on sleep. *Journal of Primary Care & Community Health, 13.*

263 Conroy, D. A., Kurth, M. E., Strong, D. R., Brower, K. J., and Stein, M. D. (2016). Marijuana use patterns and sleep among community-based young adults. *Journal of Addictive Diseases, 35*(2), 135–143.

264 See footnote 264.

that those who drank alcohol and used cannabis might also find helpful benefits from the CBT-I group.[265] This was so interesting to me because I've noticed that those who drink alcohol and use substances may struggle with the CBT-I protocol and find that treatment lasts a bit longer, but they've still seen good effects from treatment.

The verdict: My knee-jerk reaction to all of this research is that using marijuana for sleep (in general) depends on the person, how often they're taking it, and for what reason. If you're already taking medications, it's better to chat with your doctor about this because drugs interact differently with each other. We know in the case of melatonin, they sometimes put serotonin in these melatonin pills, so those who are taking an SSRI are at higher risk of complications. You might not be sure how marijuana interacts with other drugs, but a professional would know more. Another factor to consider is using it in moderation. It seems most people who chronically use marijuana have a rebound insomnia effect, which makes their sleep quality feel worse after they stop using it. If marijuana has a side effect that causes drowsiness or sleepiness, then we stop taking it. Well, we can expect to have difficulty falling or staying asleep that night.

On a personal note, I am curious about the substances I use and how they affect my sleep. If I take an OTC one night because of jet lag, I try to abstain from it the next night to avoid tolerance effects. I talk to my doctor to make sure this is the right choice for me because it may look different for other people. When in doubt, do some research, talk to your doctor, and figure out your sleep goals. Once you have a decisive goal in mind, it'll be easier to figure out whether medical marijuana or other substances are right for you.

---

265 Miller, M. B., Carpenter, R. W., Freeman, L. K., Curtis, A. F., Yurasek, A. M., and McCrae, C. S. (2022). Cannabis use as a moderator of cognitive behavioral therapy for insomnia. *Journal of Clinical Sleep Medicine, 18*(4), 1047–1054.

Chapter 6

THE IMPACT OF STRESS ON SLEEP

Ah, stress. We all have it. We all experience it differently. We all have different stressors in life. When we're stressed, we don't operate as efficiently as we do if we are in a relaxed state. I've thought a lot about stress and how it impacts sleep and remember thinking, *Do I have a sleep issue or a stress issue?* Stress contributes to poor sleep, which might influence my stress response. I can't control certain stressors in my life, but maybe I can control some of my sleep.

The crazy part is so many things are outside of our control in life. So. Many. Things. While you're here, let's talk a little more about stress, how it affects you and your sleep, and what you *can* do about it now. Basically, we're becoming curious about stress and examining how it affects us, even if there's no solution. It's the next best thing if we don't have a solution. And one quick reminder to help you get motivated to read this chapter:

Sleep won't fix it if your soul is tired.

Sleep can't fix certain stressors. When your soul is tired, it's more about finding your sense of purpose rather than sleeping it off. Sleeping might push you further away from figuring out your "why" and cause more stress. However, sometimes we need sleep when we're stressed because our body is exhausted. It's sometimes hard to know the difference.

What Is Stress?

There are so many different definitions of stress. So. Many.

Stress can be a state of mental or emotional strain or tension from very demanding circumstances. MedlinePlus says that "it can be a state of emotional or physical tension."[266] The Merriam-Webster dictionary characterizes it as "physical, chemical, or emotional factor that causes bodily or mental tension."[267] I'm sure we all have a definition of stress, but my favorite definition is from the Mental Health Foundation, which defines it as "the feeling of being overwhelmed or unable to cope with mental or emotional pressure."[268] Yeah, that one hits different.

Stress looks different for everyone, especially minorities and those with untreatable illnesses, or those who experience uncontrollable stress that influences their livelihood. For example, if we only look at binary gender categories, women tend to report lower sleep quality than men.[269] In terms of sexual orientation, bisexual and lesbian women report lower sleep quality than heterosexual women.[270] Queer Latinx/Hispanic men and women tend to report sleeping a shorter

---

266 MedlinePlus. (n.d.). *Stress and your health.* U.S. National Library of Medicine. https://medlineplus. gov/ency/article/003211.htm.

267 Merriam-Webster. (n.d.). *Stress definition & meaning.* https://www.merriam-webster.com/ dictionary/stress.

268 Mental Health Foundation. (2021). *What is stress?* https://www.mentalhealth.org.uk/a-to-z/s/stress.

269 Millar, B. M., Goedel, W. C., and Duncan, D. T. (2019). Sleep health among sexual and gender minorities. In D. T. Duncan, I. Kawachi, and S. Redline (Eds.), *The social epidemiology of sleep* (pp. 187–204). Oxford University Press.

270 See footnote 270

amount of time as compared to their heterosexual peers.[271] These are factors that are not "controllable" (a.k.a. we can't change our race or sexual identity) that tend to influence sleep. However, there may be a biological driver for stress that we mostly share as humans.

Stress: A Biological Perspective

We know that stress affects sleep, but what *actually* happens to our bodies during times of stress? I like to talk about the biological stress response, which includes our sympathetic nervous system and hypothalamic-pituitary-adrenal (HPA) axis. The goal is to give you an inside scoop into what happens to your body so that we can figure out how to incorporate sleep into this puzzle. We've already briefly talked about the first part of the stress response, which includes the arousal of our sympathetic nervous system. Here are more of the details.

The Nervous System

The sympathetic nervous system regulates our stress response (a.k.a., the fight-flight-or-freeze response), and the parasympathetic nervous system controls our relaxation response. Our sympathetic nervous system (stress response) becomes engaged when our body recognizes a stressor. This can be a bear in the woods, the idea of claiming bankruptcy, your boss voicing dissatisfaction with your work, or you not knowing when your next meal is; the list goes on and on. Your body then releases epinephrine and norepinephrine, fancy hormones that help your body prepare for battle. You might start to notice your

---

271 Trinh, M., Agénor, M., Austin, S. B., and Jackson, C. L. (2017). Health and healthcare disparities among U.S. women and men at the intersection of sexual orientation and race/ethnicity: A nationally representative cross-sectional study. *BMC Public Health, 17*(1), 964.

heart rate increase, or you might start sweating. The battle might be to run from a bear or to prepare for an uncomfortable conversation. Either way, your body is getting ready to keep you safe.

On the other hand, when we're relaxed, our parasympathetic nervous system is dominant, also known as our relaxation response. It's when you're totally vibing, not super stressed about anything. We notice that our breathing slows down, and our body engages in metabolic recovery. This helps us engage in those restorative activities, such as repairing muscles and tissue, mental reorganization, maintaining body temperature, or restoring our body's energy reserve. This is quite the opposite of what happens when we are stressed—our parasympathetic nervous system checks out and lets the sympathetic nervous system be the main character.

So, our sympathetic nervous system is engaged; what happens next? Let's start with the hypothalamic-pituitary-adrenal (HPA) axis. This sounds wild, but don't worry; we'll walk through this together. You have one of these, so you'll want to pay attention. The HPA axis represents the interaction between the hypothalamus, pituitary, and adrenal glands, which is our body's response to stress.

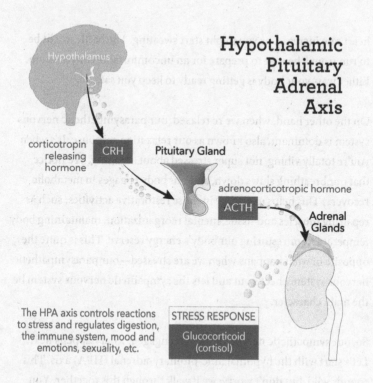

Hypothalamic Pituitary Adrenal Axis

Hypothalamus

corticotropin releasing hormone — CRH

Pituitary Gland

adrenocorticotropic hormone — ACTH

Adrenal Glands

The HPA axis controls reactions to stress and regulates digestion, the immune system, mood and emotions, sexuality, etc.

STRESS RESPONSE

Glucocorticoid (cortisol)

So, picture this. Your hypothalamus gets word that there's a stressor happening, and it starts the show. It says, "Everyone, gather around; we have some work to do." It's a cluster of nuclei in the brain that instructs the pituitary gland to release a hormone. So, the pituitary gland screams to the adrenal glands, "Hey! Start the flow!" and the adrenal glands produce steroid hormones called glucocorticoids. Let's pause; what the hell are glucocorticoids? These specific hormones are cortisol and adrenaline, also known as stress hormones. Sounds familiar, right?

Whoa, whoa. We're going too fast here. Let's back up. What happens with cortisol? Does it flow through our bloodstream on a floaty tube with a piña colada and tell our other cells that we're stressed? Does it yell out to the heart, "Go faster! We're gonna die!"? Not quite. More happens before cortisol is released into the bloodstream. It is the stress hormone, but it doesn't cause more stress; it helps the body respond to stress.

Your hypothalamus secretes corticotropin-releasing hormones (CRH) into the bloodstream, which increases sympathetic nervous system arousal. It keeps your heart rate pumping so your body is ready for anything. Eventually, the pituitary gland sees CRH and wants to level up, releasing adrenocorticotropic hormone (ACTH) into the bloodstream, too. So ACTH eventually finds the door to the adrenal glands. It binds to the doorknob of the adrenal gland door (a.k.a. the surface of the adrenal cortices), and the adrenal glands secrete glucocorticoids, one of these being cortisol.

Cortisol helps our body recognize that it needs to increase blood pressure to help your skeletal muscles prepare for physical activity. Some people end up running in this situation. Maybe you're not physically running, but maybe you're walking away from a tough conversation. If this was a vicious animal, I'm sure you'd be running for your life. Your body releases glucose, helping you have more energy to deal with stress. And, as we chatted about before, the presence of cortisol lets the body know that we don't have to worry about other things, like libido. It's kind of difficult to achieve an orgasm when your body thinks you're running away from a serial killer.

I am generalizing here, and there's more that happens in this process, but think about this happening every time we're stressed. Now think of chronic stress. The stress that never goes away, that you feel almost all of the time. Do you think your body cares about sleep when this is happening? Absolutely not. Sleep is seen as a threat because if you're sleeping, you can't defend yourself. And if you can't defend yourself, well…[insert any terrible life-or-death scenario here]. Our way of

handling or acknowledging stress can truly affect our sleep, especially
when this stress is out of our control.

Chronic HPA Axis Dysregulation Stressors

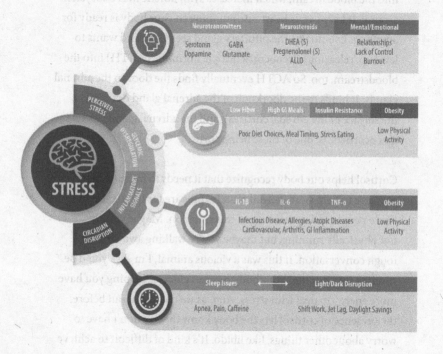

The Impact of Stress
on Insomnia

Our body is focused on surviving and maintaining homeostasis. So, if it has a stress response, it helps us gear up to deal with the stressor so that we can essentially come back to baseline (a.k.a. normal, whatever that is). Our bodies are biologically wired similarly, meaning we may have predictable ways of dealing with stress. When you hear the fight-flight-or-freeze response, I'm sure you can put yourself into one of these categories. You either fight and lean into the stress to figure it out, run away, or feel so paralyzed that you don't know what to do in stressful situations.

We know that stress impacts our ability to initiate and sometimes maintain sleep. When you're stressed or anxious, you might get into bed and notice your mind wandering. You might notice thoughts or that you're unable to feel relaxed. You might have difficulty closing your eyes because you feel like there's so much unfinished business. You might not even be responding to stress in bed, but your brain remembers the stress from earlier in the day.

Although we might have trouble falling asleep due to stress, it also impacts our ability to sleep soundly throughout the night. Cortisol, the stress hormone we talked about earlier, usually decreases as we begin our nighttime bed routine. Of course, this will look different for shift workers or those with nontraditional work schedules. If cortisol levels remain high, it is unlikely that we will sleep soundly throughout the night.[272] Our sleep issues may persist because of increased cortisol,

272 Breus, M. (2022). *Sleep and stress.* The Sleep Doctor. https://www.sleep.org/how-sleep-works/
     sleep-and-stress.

but they may also stick around because sleep issues *cause* increased cortisol. It's kind of like the chicken-or-the-egg theory—we're not sure which one comes first. To top it all off, we know that cortisol is affected when we attempt to change our body's natural rhythm for sleep, such as going to sleep or waking up in a way that doesn't align with our body's sleep-wake cycle.

We also may become more stressed knowing that we aren't getting enough sleep. You might wake up and think, "Fuck, now I'm going to be exhausted all day because I only got four hours of sleep." Well, you're right; you might be exhausted. And you are also punishing your body for something you might not be able to control. If you knew how to fix it, you would have by now.

I'm sure you experienced some sleep issues during the pandemic. I mean, shit, who didn't? I had nightmares when I learned of my friends or family contracting COVID-19. They had what everyone was fearful of, so that meant I was living in fear, too. How could I get to sleep knowing my loved one might not make it through the night? We can't expect ourselves to simply sleep through this or sleep soundly when the world around us is crumbling. The pandemic also caused a lot of changes in childcare, working from home, coexisting with your partner during work hours, limited routines, and low sleep drive due to sitting around all day. It was hard to figure out how to exist, let alone sleep well.

I see stress as a risk factor for insomnia and other sleep disorders. When we're stressed, it ignites our body in ways that inhibit our ability to initiate or maintain sleep. Handling that stress is key, but what if we don't have solutions? I'll tell you that it's important to lean in sometimes rather than avoid stress, even if you don't have solutions. Over time you may become more accustomed to handling this stress by compartmentalizing, but it's important to validate that it is real.

The Importance of Acknowledging Stress, Even If You Don't Have Solutions

Do we have solutions for every stressor out there? Absolutely not. Every person handles stress differently (i.e., stress resiliency), and we each have a different approach and perspective when it comes to stress. Some people completely ignore their stress and can fall asleep gracefully. If it's not broken, don't fix it. However, most of us live in a world where we're acknowledging gut-wrenching news almost daily, reminding us of how shitty life can be.

Identify the Uncontrollable Stressor(s)

I woke up last Friday to find that the Supreme Court had overturned Roe v. Wade. I haven't slept well since. I'm telling you, I've been waking up every few hours and it's difficult to fall back asleep. I'm sure you can think of something happening in the world that keeps you up at night. This was a similar reaction to other historical events, such as society questioning same-sex and interracial marriage, women being unable to drive in Saudi Arabia, and the injustices resulting in the deaths of George Floyd, Ahmaud Arbery, and Breonna Taylor, to name a few. I'm sure you've been here, too. These feel uncontrollable and difficult to manage because there may not be many direct solutions to take action in the present moment.

Like you, I don't want to turn off the news because I want to be informed, yet my body is begging for a break from these constant updates. I'm not sure if we were equipped as humans to handle bad news this often. However, when I gave myself a break and noticed that

I don't have a solution to fix it, but I have a solution of how I'll handle it day by day, that helped reduce my stress levels. It was tough for me to live in this gray area, but it's important because the black-and-white wasn't doing me any good. This is one example of how we can acknowledge stress that we can't control and learn to work through it. It's not ideal but it's better than weeks of sleepless nights. That doesn't help anyone.

Think about the Arrow

I like to use the arrow example to explain how stress impacts our well-being. This analogy comes from Buddhist teachings[273] and can be used to discern controllable stressors from uncontrollable ones.

The First Arrow

The stress that you experience is technically the first arrow. You got shot with an arrow unexpectedly and couldn't control that arrow. Picture that arrow as systematic racism, poverty, or a low socioeconomic status. Maybe it's a physical disability that you were born with, or that you're a woman trying to make it in a patriarchal society. You might be a nonbinary person constantly having to educate other people about your existence in hopes of validating why you're here in the first place. It's exhausting. That arrow hurts and causes a lot of pain, and you can't do much about it.

---

273 Neale, M. Buddhist origins of mindfulness meditation. In J. Loizzo, M. Neale, and E. J. Wolf (Eds.), *Advances in Contemplative Psychotherapy* (pp. 17–34). Routledge.

The Second Arrow

Then, think about all those unhelpful thoughts you have, the shame you put yourself through, the extra stress on top of the original stress—well, that's a second arrow. You might guilt yourself into a different identity because of the stress. You might avoid certain topics to make other people comfortable being in your presence. You might engage in the most horrible, critical self-talk because you think this is the only way to punish yourself for your existence. You might hate yourself because of your disability and struggle to see the good in life because you can't work past the fact that you'll never walk again. The second arrow serves as a second layer of pain and suffering. It's basically how you treat yourself and talk to yourself because of the stress.

This second arrow is where you can exhibit control. You might be able to acknowledge it at times, and it serves as another layer of pain and suffering. You're already in pain; why put yourself through more? When I think about it this way, it's easier for me to be nicer to myself. I'm kicking myself while I'm already down, and it might not be so helpful for myself or others around me.

We know that ruminating on our stress may cause issues falling asleep more than the level of stress itself. For example, if you're dealing with a tough stressful event that you can't shake, you will likely struggle to get to sleep if you persistently focus on this event. Now let's say you're dealing with lower-level stress, but you can't shake it. This may similarly affect sleep. It's not how big the stressor is but how we perceive it. Either way, the stressful event may not be something we can change, and our brains think the only way to handle it is to think about it.

Assessing for Uncontrollable Stressors

It can be hard to figure out the controllable versus uncontrollable stressors in our life. For simplicity reasons, I ask myself, "Do I have a way to reduce this stressor by 10 percent?" If the answer is yes, I try to take provisions to do this for myself or others. Maybe I try to wake up a little earlier to get more organized in the day so I'm not as overwhelmed. Or, I try to have that tough conversation and set a boundary even if it's difficult. I might not want to do these things, but it might help a little.

If this stressor is unmanageable, I try to manage my sense of self. I know that sounds weird, so I'll give you an example. You might be at a meeting with a racist, sexist, or homophobic person. I'm sure you want to punch them straight in the dome. That would probably cost you your job and then you'd have to figure out how to pay your bills. If that was the solution with no consequences, I'd say lay into them knuckle deep! In an alternate universe we could maybe do this, but right now it might not help your case. It doesn't mean their behavior isn't hurtful, but you might have to take the high road, which I know you're sick of doing by this point.

So, what do you do about this? You try to manage your sense of self. At the end of the day, you have yourself as a body, a soul, a human. I tell myself that I have somewhat of a choice of how I show up, how I choose to respond, how much eye contact I make, where I sit, how I use silence to influence the conversation, and more. These small controllables do not fix racism, sexism, or homophobia. We are thinking in the gray area, not the black-and-white.

The Second Arrow in Real Time

I was in a meeting once with a white, cisgender, heterosexual man who was probably about thirty years older than me. He had the *most* misogynistic views (he once said, "There's no place for a woman CEO") and frequently made objectifying comments to his male colleagues in front of us. They sat in silence while it happened. This silence spoke volumes for the women in the room, especially women of color because that's who he targeted the most. It was mortifying. I couldn't understand why nobody said anything to him and how they allowed this behavior. I was only at this company for a few weeks, and I could see the fear in everyone's eyes. They didn't want to lose their jobs. So I figured I'd find one of my controllables and give this a go. I had some privilege on my side, so I figured I might as well use it for good.

He kept talking over me. I started to become infuriated. I felt like I couldn't control my emotions. But those emotions are valid, so no need to challenge them. I'm in control (somewhat) of how I choose to show up (this is the second arrow). I remembered that, and as I began talking he interrupted again. I said to myself, "Kristen, girl, let's just fuck around and find out." So, I kept talking. This was my moment of control—very small, of course, but it was better than nothing. We talked over each other until a colleague intervened and said, "We can't hear either of you," and I responded with, "Yeah, it seems that someone is talking over me." It was gentle enough that he felt embarrassed rather than angry, and that's where I knew I won. I didn't want to make him feel bad, and I also wanted to take control of this stress. That battle wasn't over for a long time, but it was a start.

This is a minor example of a situation I seemingly had no control over, but I could control small parts of it, and most of that was how I showed up. (I recognize my privilege in this situation, too, because I

was only at the company for a few weeks and didn't care about losing
my job. It's important to assess this before intervening.) These types
of situations kept me up at night. I questioned myself and wondered if
women had a place in the workforce. I wondered how other men could
sit around as this happened, and I truly wondered how people like
this made it far in life. Oh, wait. What's that? Yeah, we're getting some
information from headquarters. It sounds like this was a combination
of white privilege, misogyny, and male insecurity. Got it. Makes
sense now.

You might feel small in a room full of people with more power over
you. Of course, you assess your safety before acting on these thoughts.
You might not be able to voice anything in the moment, but realizing
you can show up differently, ignore them, or dismiss their claims (in
your mind) can be helpful to regulate emotions in the moment. Of
course, accountability is key for people who dismiss our values, and
that's the main problem. Sometimes we don't have control over that,
which is the problem with the system. And this system may continue
to fail you, over and over again.

Think about this happening repeatedly, in different circumstances, for
your entire life. This is a small aspect of your control in a system that
doesn't value you or intentionally tries to marginalize you. These are
deep words, and if you're part of a minority group, you've probably
felt this.

Sometimes these stressors are hard to assess. You can't fix the entire
problem, but you might have control over a small piece and can
reduce your stress by taking control over another aspect. It might feel
counterintuitive or not worth the energy, but your inner child will
celebrate for you. Small pieces of regaining your control will help you
feel better than you did before. The stressor will still exist, and you

will too. You become more confident with every interaction and every choice to combat the stressor.

How about in Therapy?

I pull from a few different modalities to help the client handle stress within the context of insomnia, which I'll talk about in a bit. Chatting about stressors and stress-provoking thoughts is important and can be the most sensitive part of insomnia treatment, in my opinion. We're dealing with the inner workings of someone's mind, their deepest thoughts and vulnerabilities. Yep, it gets deep in insomnia treatment. It's not about fancy pillows and making yourself comfortable. But first, let's state the obvious. I'm a clinical psychologist, so we love to assess every little thing (the limit does not exist!).

We could talk about stress and chalk it up to, "We can't do anything about it, so why focus on it? Here's information on deep breathing exercises." Well, this is entirely unhelpful because it doesn't give the person a solution for their stress, even if they don't have a *big* solution, like dismantling the patriarchy. If you are going to dismantle it, by the way, I'll leave my contact information at the end of this book. I'm down to go with you on this one. Pack a bag; we ride at dawn, hunnies.

Anyway, I like to take a few sessions and explore these uncontrollables with the client. It's probably what's keeping them up at night. We can talk about all the tactics in the world, but if we can't come to terms with our stress, it'll damage our sleep health.

Here are some examples of questions that I ask. Take some time and try to come up with answers to these if they apply to you. If not, imagine how this may impact someone else's sleep. You might not think these questions apply, but I promise that stress impacts our ability to fall or stay asleep, so this is important.

One of the major questions I ask every client is, "What do you think society misunderstands about you? What do you wish that other people could understand about your experience?" Here are a few others:

- You mentioned working with a few people that aren't respectful toward you. I know we're probably putting it lightly here. Tell me about what it's like experiencing racism within the workplace. What thoughts keep you up at night? Share what you feel comfortable with.

- Tell me more about how your generation experiences stress and how that gets in the way of communicating with other generations.

- Tell me how euphoria (or lack thereof) related to your gender identity impacts how you see yourself.

- What obstacles are you trying to overcome?

- Tell me how your skin color influences how you sleep at night.

- What is it like to have your words translated by an interpreter?

- If you had a magic wand, what uncontrollables in your life would you change? Do these uncontrollables keep you up at night?

- How do you think your race or ethnicity impacts your stress and sleep?

- Are the language barriers you experience a point of stress, shame, or anxiety? Tell me about them.

- How does your religion foster connection or disconnection from the people you love?

- How has serving in the military changed your view of the world?

- What's it like walking into a room of white people at work when you're the only POC? Does it impact your sleep? In what ways? I'm all ears.

- How does your experience as a mid-fat person affect your mental and physical well-being related to sleep?

- Tell me about your cultural upbringing and how this impacts how you view the world.

- How has your sexual identity shaped the way you trust and interact with others? Does this seem like a source of stress for you?

- After you immigrated to a new country, what was your biggest fear? Tell me about your current fears today. If not, is there some resemblance to this fear that shows up in your daily interactions? What is it like?

- How do body, shape, and weight influence your sleep experience?

- What's it like being the smartest person in the room? Is it lonely?

- How does your privilege impact how you see your insomnia issues?

- The world can be a scary place right now; tell me about how this impacts your sleep. What do you wish for the world?

- How does your income level affect how you prioritize your sleep? Can you give yourself some breaks here and there? What is the cost of taking a break from your unique situation?

This isn't an exhaustive list and most of these questions don't have solutions that we can act on within the context of therapy. Yet, the answers to these questions keep people up at night. The key is that you're right; we can't fix these situations. But giving the client space to explore these issues and how they're impacted is important. The way we think about our stress is as important as utilizing stress management techniques, in my opinion.

Sometimes clients feel more empowered when they come face-to-face with the one thing that's been bothering them. If there are no viable solutions, we discuss how to manage these issues.

Protocols Used in Therapy

The original CBT-I protocol calls for assessing stress symptoms and how people cope with their issues, but I find it helpful to focus a lot of time on this area if someone experiences a lot of stress. Sometimes a client and I are working on stress rather than sleep and their sleep patterns remit once we handle some of the stressors.

Most of the time I use CBT-I in combination with another modality, such as Acceptance and Commitment Therapy (ACT), depending on the client. CBT is focused on how our emotions influence our thoughts and behaviors. Sometimes our behaviors influence our thoughts and emotions. I'm not going to dive into the entire protocol here, but part of the cognitive restructuring may be helpful for thoughts about stressors outside our control.

CBT

Using CBT can be a sticky situation because most of the time, our emotions and thoughts are valid when we think about uncontrollable stressors. We aren't trying to challenge the person's emotions but to figure out if this thought truly helps them in the moment. It can feel pretty invalidating to say, "Yep, this emotion doesn't make sense," so we want to use this modality with caution, depending on the client. It's not clinically indicated for everyone, but I'll show you how I use this to address uncontrollable stressors.

Let's take the example of someone with a physical ability issue. It might be difficult for them to get comfortable at night while in bed. They might say, "I am so frustrated, and I hate my body." They might spiral and talk to themselves critically based on this one thought. That spiral is the part we chat about changing, and it might start with that initial thought. I might say, "This emotion (frustration) is completely valid. Anyone in your situation would feel similarly. Is the thought of hating your body helpful for you to feel better or is it unhelpful and causing you to feel worse? We're not going to challenge it, but maybe we can alter it to make it more helpful." Then, I help the client come up with something more compassionate like, "I'm frustrated that my body does this every now and then when I get into bed. It doesn't mean I won't get to sleep at some point, and I'm allowed to feel this way." It is a small piece of what you can control from the situation to make life easier for you. Remember that the second arrow hurts like hell.

When my clients are struggling, I remind them of what a supervisor once told me: "All feelings are valid, but not all behaviors are." This means that we're allowed to think and feel whatever we want and how we choose to act upon these thoughts (or not) might be within our control. And there are outliers here, so it truly depends on the client. Regardless, it's a great example of how you might become curious about your thoughts at night or when you think about uncontrollable stressors.

How Parts of CBT Can Help

CBT can be helpful in becoming more mindful and curious about how thoughts influence our emotions and behaviors. It's not to challenge them all the time, although I know this is one of the core tenets of CBT.

I sometimes think about emotions and thoughts as data points to help me figure out what to do from here. I might notice a flood of thoughts and not get into bed until I "come to terms" with them, even if there's no solution. This might look like inviting the thoughts in for a while to see what's going on or pushing them away for tomorrow because it's not helpful to go down the rabbit hole. However, most clients notice they feel the best when they reduce their avoidance.

Yuck, avoidance is such a weird word, right? I'm sure it brings up some feelings. Like avoiding the gym for a few weeks or avoiding having that tough conversation with your mom. I picture my anxiety-provoking thoughts like a little bubble that sits next to me. The more I become familiar with these thoughts, the less anxiety they might produce. Thus, the bubble gets smaller over time. It doesn't impact me as much. Avoidance makes most things bigger, so it's nice to come up with a solid baseline rather than having our thoughts make things worse for us (even if they're valid and accurate).

There's a concept of thinking about our thoughts (a.k.a. metacognition). We can think about our thoughts and see how that changes our feelings or behaviors. It's not that simple when we're dealing with shit that's outside of our control; we want solutions. I like to think about the thoughts that cause the most stress, check in on them to see where they come from, and see if these thoughts are helpful. It's a spin-off of the CBT skill called "catch it, check it, change it."[274] Changing the thought may feel invalidating, so we like to assess where it comes from. Is thinking about this for a long time helping me feel better? It's normal to think about stuff for a few minutes or even an hour or two. Is that helping your mood? If there aren't many solutions,

---

274 BBC. (n.d.). *Catch it, check it, change it.* BBC Headroom Wellbeing Guide. http://downloads.bbc.
       co.uk/headroom/cbt/catch_it.pdf.

you might start to feel stuck. So, this skill helps people pull themselves out of this feeling sometimes.

ACT

What about ACT? Dr. Harris, ACT Trainer and author of *The Happiness Trap*, noted that, "the aim of ACT is to create a rich, full and meaningful life, while accepting the pain that inevitably goes with it."[275]

Well, let me start by giving you a brief, simplified version of how I use this when it comes to stress. Acceptance and Commitment Therapy (ACT) has a few core tenants, including mindfulness, acceptance, defusion, self-as-context, values, and committed action. This isn't clinically indicated for insomnia and sometimes it's helpful to see insomnia within the context of unresolved anxiety or stress that pops up at night. Okay, so all these fancy words, what do they mean?

Values

ACT doesn't necessarily target symptom reduction. It focuses on the person living a life based on their values and taking committed action toward those values. You might consider connection and relationships to be strong values, and if you're not seeing your friends as often, it might make you feel low. It's because you aren't living a life based on your established values. Ask yourself, "What do I really want out of life?" or, "If I could change anything about my life with a magic wand, what would it be?" You might be able to act based on those things

275 Harris, R. (2007). *Acceptance and commitment therapy (ACT) introductory workshop handout.* https://thehappinesstrap.com/upimages/2007%20Introductory%20ACT%20Workshop%20 Handout%20-%20%20Russ%20Harris.pdf.

you would change. You might pretend to show up as someone with confidence, just as an experiment.

Living a values-based life might reduce stress in some areas and make you feel more empowered and secure because you want to show up as someone with a sense of secure identity. You figure out what your values are, then figure out goals based on those values.[276] We notice that when people feel a sense of fulfillment in their lives, it makes it easier to handle uncontrollable stressors. So, we're not directly handling the stressors we can't change, but we're closer to living a better life.

Acceptance

Ah, this is probably the most difficult part of ACT but the most important for stress and sleep. ACT suggests that living a fulfilling life might mean acceptance of experiences that aren't within your control. I always used to get caught up on the word *acceptance*. I'd think, *So I'm just supposed to accept this and act like everything is okay?* Well, no. That wouldn't be helpful.

> **Accepting and agreeing are two separate experiences.**

You might not agree with your insomnia or that you have to deal with all of these uncontrollable stressors, and you accept that this is what you're dealing with. You are ending the war in your mind. You end the war of the struggle to find solutions. The invalidating experiences of questioning if this is really what's happening to you. It's time to

---

276 See footnote 276.

allow yourself to heal, and healing might start with acknowledging the shit you can't stand but accepting that this shit is your life. It's almost like you're leveling with yourself to say, "Yup, this is exactly what I'm dealing with." It could be very painful, which is why some people avoid this part.

It's a sobering experience and it takes a lot of practice. Another way I try to talk about acceptance is the willingness to experience uncomfortable feelings or emotions to do something in accordance with your values. An example of this might be attending a family gathering to foster the relationship you have with your sibling even though you and your parents don't get along. If you didn't see your sibling, you might be even more depressed. So, you don't have to love seeing your parents or approve of it to accept that being around them might be helpful to seeing your sibling, who brings you joy.

How do you practice acceptance of stuff that's out of your control? Well, you acknowledge the discomfort (e.g., "I can't stand how this feels"), notice the emotion (e.g., "I'm having a feeling of disappointment and sadness right now"), and allow it to be there. Sometimes allowing the experience is the part that makes us feel the most uncomfortable but the most validated. Dr. Harris suggests we may as well let something be there because, well, it's already there. We stop pushing it away, wasting energy on avoiding the topic or fighting with it. We make room for it. We invite these feelings into the room and sit with them for a while. We soften around these experiences and we allow the gray area to exist rather than the black-and-white experience of loving, accepting, and agreeing with everything. Because that isn't realistic.

Mindfulness

In addition to acceptance, ACT suggests that you be so present with
the moment that you can be open to experiencing life as it is *in* the
present moment (mindfulness). When we're truly present, we can
accurately perceive what's happening to us and how we feel about
certain situations. When we're on autopilot or distracted, it might be
difficult to acknowledge how we *truly* feel about something because
other stuff gets in the way. It's helpful to know what we're working
with. If you're not buried in your phone, you might describe where
your stressors come from or why it's difficult to fall asleep at night
because you've been thinking that people might not see who you are
since they see your chronic illness first. Not sure if you've caught on
by now, but the tenants of ACT seem to be strikingly familiar to a few
Buddhist concepts. [277]

Defusion

It's also about looking at your thoughts rather than feeling like you
are your thoughts (defusion). You notice these thoughts and see them
as data points, and you help yourself not to get caught up in them.
You might become curious about your thoughts and ask yourself, "Is
this thought an example of what I am truly experiencing, or are my
thoughts adding to my stress?" The key to defusion isn't to get rid
of these thoughts; it helps reduce unhelpful thoughts and helps the
person become more powerful than their thoughts.

On the opposite end, cognitive fusion means that we see thoughts
as true reality. It means what we are thinking about is happening in

---

277 Fung, K. (2015). Acceptance and commitment therapy: Western adoption of Buddhist tenets?
     Transcultural Psychiatry, 52(4), pp. 561-576.

real-time. You might be thinking a lot of thoughts—some that don't fully provide a true picture of what's happening at the moment—and considering them hard facts. This is where the sticky situation arises again. We don't want to invalidate our emotional experiences, and we have to acknowledge that thoughts and feelings might be different.

When we engage in defusion, we notice that thoughts may or may not be true. We don't automatically digest these thoughts as truth because they don't rule our lives. We can't follow our thoughts' advice no matter what without being curious because we might be engaging in a thought pattern that isn't so helpful. However, if you notice your thoughts and they are a true depiction of the reality you're living in, no need to challenge them. That's where acceptance comes in. Sometimes I ask myself, "Am I hooking onto these thoughts, or can I unhook myself and be an observer really quick? What would that be like?" It helps me figure out if the thought is helpful or unhelpful or if it'll help me reach my goals.

The Bottom Line

Sometimes we don't have control over certain things in life. It sucks. We wish we had solutions and wish things could be different. That wishing might be a valid experience, and it might not be realistic. So we are wishing and waiting for things to get better, and guess what? They never do. We can't wait for someone to save us, even though most of us would benefit from this.

I think our society is a tough place to live, especially given our circumstances over the past decade. It's not easy to wake up and feel completely fulfilled or that everything is fine. That's not the point. We already know it's not perfect or ideal. The key is finding small pieces you can control and glimmers of hope and fulfillment. If we don't try to do this at all, then life is entirely negative. If we do this a little, life has more flavor and balance.

Chapter 7

PUTTING IT ALL TOGETHER
Ways to Enhance the Quality of Your Sleep

So, my friends, all of our hard work has led to this. Let's summarize some ideas about how to enhance the quality of your sleep. If you're still reading, you now know about the inner workings of sleep, why we sleep, the consequences of poor sleep, the effects of medications on sleep, how sleep issues can be more than simply insomnia, and how stress impacts sleep, and the most common sleep myths. I know you can probably take all of this information and consolidate it yourself, but who wants to spend more time doing that? That's what I'm here for. Your life is probably already stressful enough, so I'll help you with this. Work smarter, not harder. :)

I won't repeat what we've talked about in earlier chapters, but I hope to combine some of this information and potentially word it differently. Sometimes that's helpful for different learning styles or perspectives.

When I think about enhancing the quality of our sleep, a few factors come to mind. I usually think about sleep drive, circadian rhythm, stress, anxiety, and how our thoughts about sleep impact our overall sleep health. Additionally, I think about the current state of the world and how the world can be a scary place. I also like to consider how the intersectionality of privilege, race, ethnicity, gender, sexuality, ability, body, shape, weight, socioeconomic status, medical conditions, and physical health influence our sleep. As you can see, there's a lot to consider.

Above all, some of these tactics won't be things you can check off a to-do list. Sometimes they require more effort to challenge ourselves in ways that we didn't expect or acknowledge that our approach to our sleep issues may be the one thing holding us back. It's almost the difference between a diet and a lifestyle change. A diet regimen is easy to identify and sometimes hard to follow through on. You figure out the things you can eat and the things you can't. You do this until you achieve your goal of enhancing your strength or increasing your movement, but you might fall back into old habits once you kick the diet. On the other hand, lifestyle changes take a lot of time and might feel like they're not making much of a difference until you look back in a few weeks and think, *Oh yeah, that did help. I didn't realize it at the time!* You don't go back to your way of life before this lifestyle change because these changes are feasible and work for your unique situation. You aren't putting yourself in a box like you would with a diet.

I always encourage my clients and readers to consider where they are personally. It's helpful to take inventory of these things before coming up with a sleep plan to figure out where to put most of your energy. If it's hard enough to prioritize sleep, we want to focus on the things that will be the best use of time. I might ask you some questions here about how you think about your culture or race, how that impacts your stress level, and how your stress impacts your sleep. You might not have all the answers. That's okay. The point is to start the conversation so that you can keep this in mind if and when you're struggling.

The most important part, in my opinion, is acknowledging the issue and coming up with small ways to enhance it. If you make it achievable, it's easier to complete. It's almost like starting a puzzle from scratch, and you add one piece per day. You won't get the whole puzzle figured out in a few days or weeks. You might have an idea of what puzzle piece you'll pick next, but focusing on each puzzle piece rather than the entire puzzle is a little more worthwhile. What this means: stick with some small steps, don't worry so much about the outcome, and focus more on your day-to-day rather than the end destination.

Managing Sleep Expectations

In an earlier chapter we talked about being a slight fuck-up and not being perfect and having realistic expectations for our sleep. Well, we aren't perfect because perfection doesn't exist. Some things you may not be able to change about your sleep. That being said, it's helpful to have realistic sleep expectations based on your body's unique needs. This involves noticing what you're doing well and what you need to improve.

Step One: Acknowledge
What You're Doing Well

We sometimes can't change our situation, but we can change some stuff around the situation. This is what we talked about in the stress chapter. I know you're thinking, *What's the point?* Well, the point is that any little step in the right direction has the potential to change our entire life or outlook, probably not in the way you intended, but it can still help in small ways. Black-and-white thinking can be helpful for certain things, like figuring out how to escape a toxic work environment or relationship. Seeing the gray area will likely help you rationalize staying in these situations. However, the gray area for sleep is helpful at times. Maybe you don't get a full eight or nine hours of sleep, but you get seven consolidated hours of sleep.

If we only focus on what's going wrong, we don't have an accurate depiction of our progress. Then we are working harder, not smarter. We're putting in all this effort when we recognize the parts that are going well, all while hating that it's not perfect. You're allowed to hate this stuff and be angry. That's the difference between accepting and agreeing. This will serve you well when talking about making changes to your sleep.

So, if you can come up with some ideas of what's going well, that's a great start. Maybe you have a solid bedtime routine or you don't wake up throughout the night. You might be excited to get more sleep or see it as self-care. Here are some ideas if you're struggling. They might not all apply, so acknowledge the ones that apply to you:

- I'm genuinely excited to start working on my sleep, although it scares me.

- I don't have many unhelpful thoughts about sleep.

- I find it easy to put my mind to rest at night.

- I don't wake up that often throughout the night (e.g., less than three times per night).

- I have a comfortable bed.

- My bedroom is dark and cool at night.

- I limit electronics before bedtime.

- I'm not excited about working on my sleep but know it can be good for me.

- I'm noticing that getting better sleep starts with small steps, kind of like reading this book.

- I don't use substances to initiate sleep at night.

- Insert your own here: _____

Step Two: Identify Your Growth Edges

Now for the stuff that makes us not-so-perfect. It's okay. We all have growth edges. I specialize in insomnia, and I still have stuff to work on sleep-wise. Our bodies change over time, so we might have to reassess our sleep health every few years.

As a reminder, accepting means you acknowledge your baseline and you aren't sugarcoating anything. Accepting does not mean you agree with it. You can accept your body struggles to wind down at night while hating that this happens. Or you might be scared to try something new. Maybe you're scared that you aren't getting enough sleep and that's holding you back from doing anything about it. Well, you can make these sleep changes even if you're afraid. "But how does that work?" I'm simplifying it here, but you know what you have to do, even if you don't want to. You just have to "do it scared."

We know what we're doing well; what do we have to work on? Make lists of what you might need help with so you can find solutions. If you don't have viable solutions, we might have to come to terms with them (like we talked about in the stress chapter). Here are a few ideas:

- I struggle with initiating sleep at night.
- I'm not sure how to set up my bedroom for the ideal sleeping situation.
- I have unhelpful thoughts about sleep that make my anxiety worse.
- I have uncontrollable stressors that I'm not sure what to do with.
- I snore or have a bed partner that snores.
- My kids/pets wake me up in the middle of the night.
- I'm afraid of taking action to help my sleep health.

- I don't think I'm worthy of sleeping well.
- Insert your own: _____

You got this!

Step Three: Focus on the Data

The more we document our struggles and victories, the easier growth becomes. We aren't all the best historians and sometimes we see things from an overly positive or negative perspective, which doesn't help us figure out what to do next. Completing a sleep diary will be helpful. You won't have to do this forever, and it'll help you gather some baseline data to either work on some strategies to help your sleep or give this to your provider so you can work through it together.

We'll talk about wake times and bedtimes in this chapter, as they vary for every person. No two people that I've seen in sleep treatment are the same. It's wild how unique we are, but we all have the same underlying sleep needs (within reason, as some of us have medical issues). "How do I figure out how much sleep I need?" Well, my answer is usually "speak with your doctor" and "search for the recommended ranges for your age group from reputable sources, like the National Sleep Foundation," but we can get the ball rolling by doing some reflection on your sleep patterns.

Take some data on your sleep. Completing a sleep diary immediately upon waking is the most helpful, and we use a detailed one for CBT-I treatment. Keep in mind that writing things down is easier than referencing your memory on your sleep patterns, so doing this daily will be the most effective. Here are some data points to consider. I took most of this from the traditional CBT-I sleep diary and added in stuff about stress and energy levels that can be important:

- Describe your bedtime routine:

  - Number of naps (and how long they lasted)

  - The time you got into bed

  - The time you attempted to fall asleep (take a guess if looking at the clock will increase anxiety)

  - How long it took you to fall asleep (I usually average this in fifteen-minute intervals, such as fifteen minutes, thirty minutes, forty-five minutes, etc.)

  - Number of awakenings

  - Duration of these awakenings

  - The time you woke up

  - The time you got out of bed

  - Amount of caffeine ingested

  - Minutes of exercise (e.g., fifteen-minute walk; thirty-minute run; ten-minute stretching session)

  - If you took any medications (prescription, over the counter, cannabis, or exogenous melatonin)

- Reflect on your energy level throughout the day. Do you feel energized? Think about what we discussed about tiredness versus sleepiness. Did you feel like you were nodding off throughout the day?

- What stressed you out today? Was it in your control or not?

- What do you wish you could change about this day?

Sleep Habit Tracker

Date	Sun	Mon	Tus	Wed	Thu	Fri	Sat
# of naps							
Duration of naps (total, in minutes)							
Time you got into bed							
Time you attempted to fall asleep							
How long it took you to fall asleep							
# of awakenings							
Duration of these awakenings							
Time you wake up							
Time you got out of bed							
Amount of caffeine ingested							
Minutes of exercise							
Medications							
What stressed you out today?							
What would you change about today?							

We have a solid idea of where to go from here when we gather some baseline data and keep tracking this information. You might not love doing this, but it will help you make more informed and intentional choices for your sleep health and life. You might find that on the days you drink more caffeine you don't sleep well, or you sleep the best when you achieve walking five thousand steps throughout the day. It will vary from person to person.

Control and Validation

Now that we've discussed some expectations, let's chat about control issues. If the word *control* triggers you, it might be a sign to lean in. This is probably one of the most important steps, in my opinion. It's acknowledging that we cannot control a lot of things in life, and these factors can cause intense pain or suffering. Even if we try every tip to enhance the quality of our sleep, we still might struggle with these things. Let's start with calling a spade a spade: there are some that are outside of your control. They're shitty things that you wish didn't exist or that you wish you could change but can't. It might bring on added stress, as we talked about earlier.

We can't control our genetics or certain life events that happen to us. However, we can control certain behavioral patterns that we engage in that make sleep worse.[278] If we don't acknowledge the non-controllables, you might still feel unsatisfied with your sleep (and your life). You don't choose where you come from, but you can make slight changes about where you go from here. Those slight changes are so incredibly important for sleep health and make a huge difference,

278 Perlis, M., Shaw, P. J., Cano, G., and Espie, C. (2011). Models of insomnia. In M. H. Kryger, T. Roth, and W. C. Dement (Eds.), *Principles and practice of sleep medicine* (5th ed.), 850–850. Elsevier.

and I'll show you why and how to do them. Have you ever heard the phrase, "work smarter, not harder"? Well, this is what I mean. We don't have to work harder to get better sleep. We can be more intentional about incorporating certain activities into our lives (or getting rid of a few), and accepting things that are outside our control. That will ultimately help us sleep better.

Sleep is usually last on the list of priorities for someone trying to survive. But sleep affects us so deeply and might help other symptoms, such as depression and anxiety. It might help our bodies function at a different capacity. It might give us a sense of esteem knowing that we can get a few hours of restoration for the next day. Sleep health (in my humble opinion) is one of the most underrated life factors that can change how we function, interact with others, and fit into certain systems that keep us stuck. When we think more clearly, we have clearer goals. If we have defined goals, it's easier to navigate life because we know where we're going.

Of course, sleep doesn't fix *the* problem. Sometimes there are no solutions to problems, which humans hate. We want solutions, and we want to feel like we are taking action toward making our problems go away.

Sleep doesn't fix if your soul is tired.

Sleep doesn't fix the body you were born with.

Sleep doesn't fix the middle-class experience of working until you retire and to barely make ends meet.

It doesn't fix how people view you, or if you are seen as valuable in life.

It doesn't fix misogyny and gender pay inequality.

It doesn't enable you to work five jobs at once to pay the bills.

It doesn't address ageism and how people aren't celebrated as they progress along their lifespans.

It doesn't fix white privilege and/or the systems that promote white supremacy.

It doesn't erase your past traumas and how those traumas have shaped you as a human.

It doesn't make someone treat you better.

It doesn't make people love you.

It doesn't make you love yourself.

Sleep doesn't fix a lot of things. However, it can help your body function better despite all these things happening. It might be the one thing that you can somewhat control in life. It's important to acknowledge the systems that keep people in the rat race. You might not have the means to change certain life experiences right now. You might not be able to quit that job that's making you miserable or avoid microaggressions that you experience daily. Being a functioning human is quite difficult when you notice everything that happens to us. And for empaths and deep thinkers, this is even more prominent. So, for someone to blindly tell you, "Hey, focus on your sleep and ignore all these other things," would be a disservice. Okay, so what do we do about the things we can't control?

We have to lean into these experiences, do what we can to make changes, and (as a last resort) accept that life is difficult at times. You don't have to agree with how life is going. In fact, you can hate every minute of it. Acknowledging this is almost like validating yourself. "Yep, this sucks, and I can't do anything about it." Acceptance provides relief, knowing that you cannot control it, and it relieves you of a little responsibility in pushing for further change.

Journaling, with Some Spice

Yuck, you might hate the word *journaling*. What's the point? I hated journaling until I had a client who kept a journal for years. They would replace their journal each year with a new one and document their thoughts every day. They didn't write novels each day but limited it to about three sentences. They spoke about the things that were the most stressful, things they were proud of, and things they were grateful for. They had balance with this, so it wasn't all negative.

We were able to reflect on these journals over the past few years and we noticed so much growth that even a therapist wouldn't catch at first glance. We might remember certain things and get rid of other things because our brains don't think we need them. It doesn't happen all the time, but it's nice to have documentation that happened in real time.

We know stress has the potential to create variations in our sleep health. What exactly stressed you out today? Think deeply about what you didn't experience in real-time but did weigh on you. Is it that you wish you were born in a different body? You notice people looking at you? You notice people aren't looking at you at all? Do you feel invisible? Do you feel too seen? Whatever it is, write it down because it's your experience and it's important. You might start to notice patterns and how they impact your life or sleep health. You might also find some solutions for these issues if you're sick of writing them down, or you might accept that they might never go away because they're a part of your life now.

How We Think about Sleep Matters

Our thoughts have the potential to influence our entire life. Sometimes these thoughts influence our feelings and behaviors, even if we don't control our thoughts. We have thousands of thoughts every day so it would be hard to control all of them. However, it might be helpful to become curious and aware of how these thoughts influence us.

I'm not asking you to change these thoughts and feelings. Most of the time they're valid and necessary to engage in problem-solving and find solutions for our issues. Ready for a buzzkill? Sometimes, there are no solutions. Big yikes. Now what? Well, your one choice point is how you think about these thoughts and feelings.

Sometimes people struggle to challenge themselves and become curious about their thoughts because they think it means avoiding feelings or invalidating themselves. "Well, if I try to feel differently about this, then I overlook that this is difficult for me." Well, you're right. The point isn't to change your feelings; those might change naturally over time. You are ending the war in your mind, the struggle to hold onto these thoughts and change your situation, because you don't have any solutions.

Exercise: Rerouting Your Thoughts

You might think that your sleep sucks and that it's hard to get to sleep. You're right. Now what? We can either act on this or challenge these thoughts. Here's a broad example of a dialogue that might happen in therapy:

Client: I hate sleep. I can never get to sleep quickly, and I always wake up exhausted.

Therapist: It's hard to even want to prioritize sleep health if it sucks all around.

Client: Yeah, for real. Like, I can't even figure out why I can't sleep well.

Therapist: But you know for sure you aren't sleeping well.

Client: Yep. So even if I change my thoughts, I won't believe them.

Therapist: Makes sense because you've been dealing with this for so long, so it seems like an impossible task to change your thoughts.

Client: Exactly. If I've been thinking this way for a long time, it must mean these thoughts are true.

Therapist: Part of this is probably true. Maybe not the entire thought. Let's get curious about the following thought: "I hate sleep. I can never get to sleep quickly, and I always wake up exhausted." Do you hate sleep, or are you uncomfortable with figuring out how to make sleep better? If you look back, are there moments in your life when it was easier to fall asleep and wake up rested?

Client: Well, I don't want to admit this, but I think you're right. I hate that I can't sleep well; I don't hate sleep itself. But that doesn't make it better.

Therapist: Of course, I'm with you there.

Client: What's the point of challenging and being curious here though? It's not going to automatically make me fall asleep quicker tonight.

Therapist: There might not be a direct connection between challenging your thoughts and sleeping soundly. Think of it like baking a cake. This ingredient helps the overall outcome of your cake. If you didn't have it, you could still eat the cake, but it might not be as good. All the ingredients are important. So, if you work on small parts of your sleep health over time, the overall picture changes.

Client: Oh, I see what you mean now. This is one important piece that will help, but this one thing alone might not help.

Therapist: Yes, somewhat. So, this might help you a lot. You might focus more on the thoughts rather than the behavioral interventions we discuss. For someone else, the behavioral interventions might work more than the thoughts because they didn't struggle in this area.

Client: Ah, I see now. So, when you asked me last session, "Is this thought helpful?" you're trying to figure out the purpose of these thoughts and see how they make it easier to sleep, right?

Therapist: Exactly! These subtle ways of being curious about your thoughts are helpful because you create room to hate parts about sleep and feel neutral about other parts. Then, you reduce the stress from your thoughts because this might be one thing you can control.

Client: True. Maybe I hate that sleep is an issue for me, but I recognize that sleep is important. Maybe that's why it's hard for me.

Therapist: I love your thought process here. It's all about balance. Now you have more room to figure out where to go from here. If you operate from the blanket statement of "I hate sleep," it reduces your ability to work on other areas of sleep or work on sleep at all. Tell me now exactly what you hate about sleep, and what you don't hate about sleep.

Client: Well, I hate that it doesn't happen naturally for me like it does everyone else. I hate that I have to focus so intensely on making it work. And the parts that I don't hate about sleep... Well, even though I struggle with sleep, I see that it's helpful for me to operate the next day. It helps me have some energy to function even though I wish I had more energy.

Therapist: I know this is hard because your initial thought of "I hate sleep" is validating. What if I told you that sleep doesn't come naturally to everybody? When we use extremes like "always" or "everyone," we distance ourselves from other people who also struggle with sleep.

Client: Exactly, I want to hate it so I feel validated, but there are also other people who struggle with sleep. I can see that for sure.

Therapist: Do you still feel validated with the newer thoughts after a curious attitude?

Client: Yes, it's just not as satisfying.

Therapist: Makes sense. I see where you're coming from. You're still allowed to hate it, honestly. I don't blame you. Which thought is more helpful for you to feel empowered to make changes: "I hate sleep" or "I hate the fact that I can't sleep well, but I don't hate sleep itself"?

Client: The second one. But if I start working on my sleep, I don't want myself to think it's not hard, and I don't want other people to think I don't still struggle with it.

Therapist: Both can be true. You can actively work on your sleep to make it better and struggle so much.

Client: Well, what do I do next? I feel like I can tackle this now.

***

This is based on true stories from a few of my clients. I changed some wording and the actual struggle, but this is a common experience. We might not want to challenge or be curious about our thoughts. This stuckness and avoidance don't help us much. When we lean in and look at these thoughts, we realize that sometimes they're unhelpful even though they're satisfying.

It's like arguing with your partner or mother. The way you say stuff matters. If you say, "I hate you," it's different than, "I hate how you talk to me when you're upset." Hate feels like a strong word, but it's a little more specific, so the person knows how to change or fix it.

Prioritizing Sleep as an Essential Function

If we think sleep isn't important and don't want to prioritize it, well, we won't. This thought essentially becomes our reality. However, if we notice our thoughts as data points and observe them without becoming entangled in them, this can be incredibly helpful. We notice when a thought is helpful or unhelpful, or if it's getting us closer to sleeping or living our best life. Sometimes we want to think certain thoughts even though we know they aren't good for us. Most of the time this happens when we are trying to validate our experience.

We might hate our situation and say, "Damn, I wish life was different." Valid. Totally makes sense. This is your way of validating the fact that this shit is *rough*. Adding onto this thought might make it a little more helpful. "Damn, I wish life was different, and I'm making changes within my control."

Basic Sleep Hygiene, but Make It Unique

Sleep hygiene is a Google search at this point, but important to cover here. I like to call it "sleep wellness strategies" rather than hygiene. It seems more approachable this way. Sleep wellness strategies help us create an environment or routine that helps us get to sleep or maintain sleep. There's a bit of nuance here. If it's not broken, don't fix it.

But if you know it *is* broken and you need to fix it but don't want to… well, let's lean into this a little. You might not want to put your phone away before bed, but you know it's helpful. Guess what? That's a choice point you'll have to make. Either stay up on social media all night and drive yourself into a downward spiral of emotions or put your phone away, be bored for a little, sit with your thoughts, and eventually fall asleep. I wish it were that easy, but you catch my drift.

On the other hand, if you're the type of person who isn't impacted by blue light or input from your phone, you might be able to continue using this strategy. If you're reading this book, I can almost assume that you're the type that becomes a little anxious when you read certain headlines or see certain types of content online. That's okay; welcome to the club.

The intention here is to make these strategies work for your situation. We might want to wake up at the same time each day, but that's not possible. You might have to modify this. I'll show you how to take basic sleep wellness strategies and formulate them into something that will work for your unique needs. I won't talk about every sleep wellness strategy here because you can do a Google search. I'll focus on the most important ones, the ones that have the potential to make or break our sleep cycles.

Consistent Wake Time

Yeah, this isn't possible for everyone. Let's be real, though. Is it possible for you but you don't like doing it? Or do you have a shift-work schedule that changes every day, making it impossible to do this?

If the latter applies to you, you will have to make a modification. If you simply don't want to, let's lean into that. How important is your sleep health? Isn't it time to show up as an ideal version of yourself? Shed those prior layers of your identity that don't apply anymore, like doing shit that makes you feel worse? I know this sounds harsh, but we might need to hear it. I know I did at one point.

We sometimes can't control our bedtime. In fact, it might be unhelpful to come up with a bedtime because so many things can get in the way of getting to sleep quickly. You might be exhausted but super anxious about something going on in your life. Or maybe you had a pain flareup. Or maybe you want to attend a protest next week, but you're scared. You might be thinking about a ton of things, and it's not helpful to simply say, "I'm going to fall asleep at nine o'clock." It's not realistic. But as we have been learning, we simply have to try and influence the factors we *can* control.

It Starts with the Earliest Bedtime

You might implement an *earliest* bedtime, which is what we do when we follow the CBT-I protocol. This means that you come up with a time to get into bed *if* you're feeling sleepy. Keyword: *if*. I figure out this number by taking an average of the hours I'm sleeping and counting backward from my wake time. I try to cap this number at six as a minimum so that I don't reduce my bed window or limit my chances of sleeping. This will depend on your specific situation, so definitely run this by your healthcare provider before implementing this.

Here's an example. If I have a wake time of six o'clock and I count back six hours, that leaves my earliest bedtime at midnight. I'm sure you're shocked. "But the earlier I get into bed the more time I have to get sleepy." I know this feels right, but it might not be the most helpful. So you only get into bed when you feel those internal cues of sleepiness (e.g., nodding off, unable to stay awake). If you're simply tired, it's helpful to engage in relaxing and mindfulness activities.

I usually give myself a thirty-minute buffer for some wiggle room, so I might make my earliest bedtime at eleven thirty. This is essential if you want consolidated sleep at night. If you're napping throughout the day, you might revise this to best match your experience.

Alternatives

If you can't wake up at the same time each day, you might have to get creative. I love this creative process when I work with clients; it's like a puzzle. If you can, try to find consistency in anything else you do. Maybe it's choosing the same shift on each day of the week. For example, maybe you can choose a shift of seven in the morning to seven at night from Monday through Wednesday and then the night shift from Thursday through Saturday. If you have this same schedule each week, it'll help with consistency. Then, you create an earliest bedtime schedule based on your shift. This might also spark some thoughts about being more intentional with your schedule. You might be hesitant to pick up shifts that have the potential to wreck your consistent sleep cycle. Sometimes we don't have a choice. If you do, it might be helpful to consider your sleep needs.

If you can't choose your shift, you might get more creative. Is there a way to work with the same crew for a few days in a row? This consistency usually reduces stress because you know what to expect. If you know what to expect, your brain won't struggle to find solutions to make life easier. You might pack your lunch and eat similar meals each day. Knowing what to expect reduces the unknown experiences that cause extra stress for your body and mind. Whenever we talk about these wellness strategies, you might say, "This doesn't apply." That's perfectly okay; you're unique. How *can* it apply? What can we modify to make it work for you?

Sleep Routine

Not everyone can create time in their schedule for a bedtime routine. Ideally, we would love thirty to sixty minutes as a wind-down period. If you come home from work and jump right into bed, you might want to think about how you can wind down *before* jumping in. Is there a way to begin your bedtime routine on your commute home from work? Sounds weird, but it might help you get to sleep faster.

If we put ourselves in the mindset that we are relaxed, focusing on sleep, and becoming excited about winding down, our bodies will agree. Our bodies might start to wind down as our minds start to relax. If you have a thirty-minute commute back to your house, you might not call your friend who rants about her abusive partner. You might not listen to crime podcasts or have that tough conversation with a coworker about how they hurt you with their words in a meeting from earlier.

We might only have time for these conversations during our drive home and that's okay. It's about being intentional with doing this every day and knowing how it may impact our sleep. I barely had enough time to come home, shower, brush my teeth, put lotion on my face, and hop into bed after my workday. I started my bedtime routine the minute I left the hospital. I would get into my car and change into my slippers (yes, I kept slippers in my car). I used makeup remover wipes to take my makeup off, so I felt a little more comfortable for the drive. It was almost like I was wiping the day off so I could transition to the next activity (usually sleep).

If you have the time and availability in your schedule to implement a solid bedtime routine, do it. I usually turn down all the lights and have invested in a few nightlights around my house. I put my phone in sleep focus mode and turn the temperature down to create a cool home environment. I put on light meditation music, usually on a timer so I don't have to worry about turning it off. I only seek out certain hashtags or follow certain accounts that bring me joy, such as puppies or baby elephants running around (it's worth a search, super cute stuff).

Handling Stress Before You Settle in to Sleep

I know these things will help me get to sleep and won't cause more anxiety. Here are a few things that I avoid at this time: difficult conversations with my partner, looking at finances, finishing my notes, calling colleagues or clients, anything work-related, uncomfortable text messages with friends, worrying about the next day. (I try to take each day as it comes so I don't spend more time thinking about it. Your job isn't paying you to worry, so you're really working and not getting paid for it.)

Most importantly, I try to handle all my stress before I walk into my bedroom. I almost see my bedroom as this sanctuary that helps with relaxation and sleep. This association is helpful because we might believe it and it may help reduce anxiety and elicit relaxation. There are many uncontrollable stressors, so ending the war in your mind before getting into bed will be helpful.

An additional measure that's super helpful for people is coming up with a bedtime routine for the days you work and the days you're home. Then, stick to this as much as you can. For some people, this routine may cause more anxiety, so we have to do an assessment to ensure this is helpful. You might reduce the steps in your routine if it feels overwhelming. I have a few clients who simply come home, shower, eat, and hop into bed and that seems to work for them.

Assessing Your Bedroom

What is in your bedroom? Does it help with sleep or relaxation? I know it's a weird question but it's helpful to do an inventory of your bedroom. If you have your own bedroom, it's worth it. I often ask people, "What is your bedroom like? What's the vibe?" If they say, "Stressful," we figure out what items are needed and what items we can take away. For example, I removed most of the overhead lights (I don't use mine) and found string lights that I turn on at night. It's not helpful to see, but it does help set the mood.

Anything in your bedroom that doesn't help with sleep can go. Okay, not so fast. Let's be intentional about this. Some things can stay if we have a solid rationale for them. Clothing and laundry make sense, but making sure this space is clean is super helpful. I notice that many people clean the rest of their house, and they leave their bedroom a wreck because, "I just sleep in it, who cares?" Your brain does. It picks up on these things, even if you're not consciously aware.

If your bedroom is a wreck with trash and clothes everywhere, it might be helpful to start by cleaning up. Put things in their place so you know what you're working with. Then, assess what you need and don't need. For most people, things that aren't helpful to have in the bedroom include: a television, anything financial or work related, anything

bright or stressful (e.g., lights, posters that provoke anxiety, pictures
that bring up unwanted memories). You don't have to get rid of these
things. They just might have a home in another room.

Knowing When to Seek Help

You might be trying your best to work on your sleep and you're
still struggling. Maybe you've seen what you're doing well, and it
still doesn't feel good enough. Maybe you feel like you're missing
something. You're not a failure; you're a human with needs. It might
be time to reach out for some help or support. A few CBT-I providers
focus solely on sleep. Finding someone who's licensed in your state is a
good place to start.

If you can't find someone who specializes in insomnia but you
have comorbid conditions, like anxiety, depression, or PTSD, your
insomnia symptoms might remit as you engage in treatment for your
other issues. Your insomnia might be part of another diagnosis, so
working on these symptoms may help your overall sleep health.

Mental health treatment might not be accessible. Maybe you don't
have insurance or can't afford a copay. This information might be
all you have. A few other good resources include the National Sleep
Foundation and the Academy of Sleep Medicine. You can follow them
on social media, and they have a great deal of information about sleep
and online resources. However, this isn't a replacement for therapy if
you're struggling.

KEEP IN TOUCH

This is where we part ways, my friends. It's been real. I'm so happy to have you on this journey and thank you for trusting me with your sleep health. You're a unique individual with specific needs, and sleep falls into this category. I hope this book helped you regain some focus on your sleep needs and wellness so you can live a more restful life. Working on your sleep health not only helps you but helps the rest of the world achieve a bit more peace.

You can follow me on social media, and we can become friends. You can find me @drkristencasey on TikTok, Instagram, and Twitter.

ADDITIONAL RESOURCES

American Academy of Sleep Medicine. (n.d.). www.aasm.org/

Newsom, R., and Dimitriu, A. (2022). *Cognitive behavioral therapy for insomnia (CBT-I)*. Sleep Foundationwww.sleepfoundation.org/insomnia/treatment/cognitive-behavioral-therapy-insomnia

Sleep Foundation. (n.d.). www.sleepfoundation.org/

Walker, M. (2017). *Why we sleep: Unlocking the power of sleep and dreams*. Simon and Schuster.

ABOUT THE AUTHOR

Dr. Kristen Casey is a licensed clinical psychologist and insomnia specialist. She was born and raised in New York City and New Jersey, where she came face-to-face with her insomnia. She's the founder and owner of two mental health companies and was an EMT for five years before becoming a psychologist. She's been featured in *Forbes*, POPSUGAR, Yahoo, *Bustle*, HuffPost, *Outside Magazine*, Livestrong, and Sleepopolis for discussing sleep and anxiety-related issues. She's most known for providing evidence-based health and wellness content about sleep and insomnia in authentic, relatable, and funny ways. The main goal of her platform is to enhance awareness of sleep health in digestible ways, and to help people feel less alone as they navigate their sleep struggles. Dr. Casey also focuses on helping therapists become their authentic selves behind the chair, all while remaining professional, helpful, and ethical. Dr. Casey strongly desires to connect with others and truly wants to see the world change for the better. She believes that taking small steps toward better sleep health can make all the difference because there's a lot that we can't control in life.

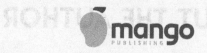

Mango Publishing, established in 2014, publishes an eclectic list of books by diverse authors—both new and established voices—on topics ranging from business, personal growth, women's empowerment, LGBTQ+ studies, health, and spirituality to history, popular culture, time management, decluttering, lifestyle, mental wellness, aging, and sustainable living. We were named 2019 *and* 2020's #1 fastest-growing independent publisher by *Publishers Weekly*. Our success is driven by our main goal, which is to publish high-quality books that will entertain readers as well as make a positive difference in their lives.

Our readers are our most important resource; we value your input, suggestions, and ideas. We'd love to hear from you—after all, we are publishing books for you!

Please stay in touch with us and follow us at:

Facebook: Mango Publishing
Twitter: @MangoPublishing
Instagram: @MangoPublishing
LinkedIn: Mango Publishing
Pinterest: Mango Publishing
Newsletter: mangopublishinggroup.com/newsletter

Join us on Mango's journey to reinvent publishing, one book at a time.